COMMUNICABLE

DAVID ALLEN &
MODERN INFECTIOUS DISEASES IN SINGAPORE

COMMUNICABLE

DAVID ALLEN &
MODERN INFECTIOUS DISEASES IN SINGAPORE

Nicholas Ngiam
Gabriel Yan
National University Hospital, Singapore

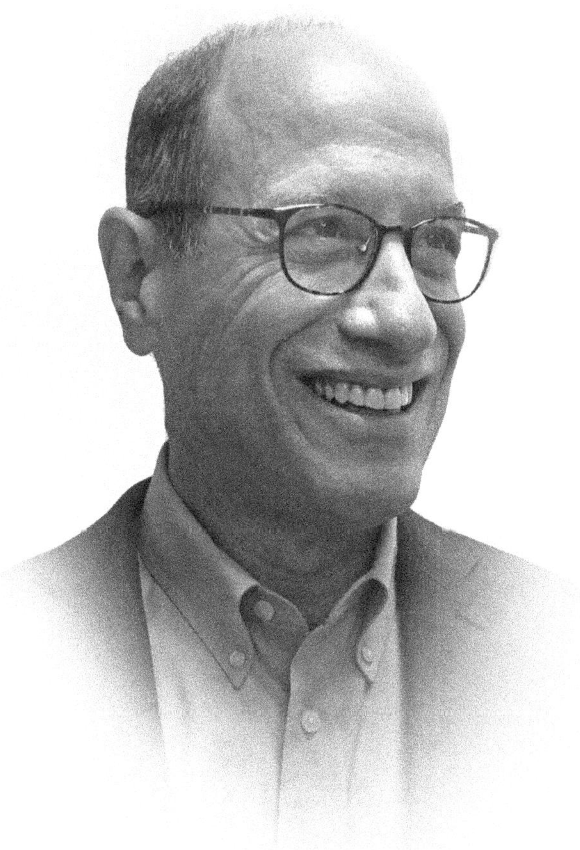

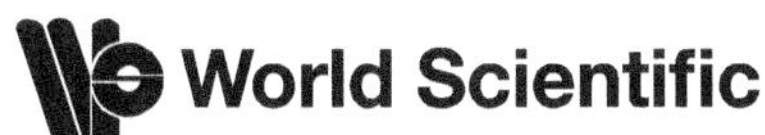

NEW JERSEY · LONDON · SINGAPORE · BEIJING · SHANGHAI · TAIPEI · CHENNAI

Published by

World Scientific Publishing Co. Pte. Ltd.

5 Toh Tuck Link, Singapore 596224

USA office: 27 Warren Street, Suite 401-402, Hackensack, NJ 07601

UK office: 57 Shelton Street, Covent Garden, London WC2H 9HE

British Library Cataloguing-in-Publication Data
A catalogue record for this book is available from the British Library.

COMMUNICABLE
David Allen and Modern Infectious Diseases in Singapore

ISBN 978-981-98-0833-5 (hardcover)
ISBN 978-981-98-0936-3 (paperback)
ISBN 978-981-98-0834-2 (ebook for institutions)
ISBN 978-981-98-0835-9 (ebook for individuals)

For any available supplementary material, please visit
https://www.worldscientific.com/worldscibooks/10.1142/14187#t=suppl

Typeset by Stallion Press
Email: enquiries@stallionpress.com

I have known David for decades and am privileged to be a member of his first group of pioneer trainees in Infectious Diseases. This book brings back fond memories of how the specialty of Infectious Diseases was recognised under his leadership. Through an "in-depth" dissection of his humorous way of putting across his thoughts, beliefs, and philosophy in nurturing young doctors and practicing medicine, this book will no-doubt influence generations of Infectious Diseases doctors for years to come.

LEO YEE-SIN, MBBS, MRCP, M.MED
Senior Consultant, National Centre for Infectious Diseases
Professor, Lee Kong Chian School of Medicine,
Nanyang Technological University
Professor, Saw Swee Hock School of Public Health,
National University of Singapore

* * *

Authors, Gabriel Yan and Nicholas Ngiam, have crafted a compelling narrative that intertwines the personal journey of David Allen and his profound impact on the field of Infectious Diseases in "Communicable: David Allen and Modern Infectious Diseases in Singapore." Beyond chronicling David Allen's journey and paying tribute to his contributions, this book provides critical insights into the evolving landscape of infectious diseases and the challenges faced by medical practitioners today and in the near future.

Former Intel CEO Andy Grove remarked that, "Bad companies are destroyed by crises; good companies survive them; great companies are improved by them". This book encourages all of us in the health profession to reflect on past practices, particularly our experiences during COVID-19, and to channel those learnings into tangible actions that can help empower the next generation of healthcare professionals to tackle future challenges, including new pandemics.

David underscores the importance of mentorship, the instilling of resilience and adaptability, being "comfortably uncomfortable" alongside a forward-thinking approach. This philosophy resonates with how NUS

Yong Loo Lin School of Medicine trains our students. We believe aspiring doctors will need to appreciate the influence of social determinants on health, be guided by scientific evidence, engage in critical thinking and inquiry, adopt a global mindset regarding existential challenges impacting global health, and lastly, possess an attitude of humility.

Doctors must "first, do good for humanity" — valuing humility, inquiry and solidarity to ensure the well-being and survival of our species.

I wholeheartedly recommend "Communicable" to everyone in the medical community. It provides inspiration and practical insights for anyone looking to shape the future of health and healthcare.

CHONG YAP SENG, MBBS, M.MED (O&G), FAMS (O&G), MD
Lien Ying Chow Professor in Medicine
Dean, National University of Singapore
Yong Loo Lin School of Medicine

* * *

In the final chapter of *Communicable*, David Allen provides wonderful advice for all of us who have the privilege of being medical doctors, either newly graduated or seasoned clinicians. He reminds us to realise each day what an exceptional life society allows us to lead as doctors. It is clear from reading this book that David lives by these words, and is doing an excellent job of sharing his daily knowledge with those who have met him in Singapore and elsewhere.

DAVID L HEYMANN, MD
Professor, Infectious Disease Epidemiology,
London School of Hygiene and Tropical Medicine, and
former visiting professor, Saw Swee Hock School of Public Health,
National University of Singapore

* * *

Every junior doctor evolves into a fusion of traits they have witnessed in or experienced from their mentors and supervisors during their formative years in training. This book recognises David's influence on the authors, where they observe nimble and original thinking, and optimism yet realism with a regular dose of humour. Admittedly, the humour is not always understood initially!

Coming out through the book is how David appreciates that he almost invariably has something to bring to the table, and in knowing this and identifying his role (perhaps personal obligation) to be helpful, he is a person who says yes to requests. Once committed, he delivers — and with quality and a smile. This book encourages us to self-reflect and consider whether we can improve, whatever stage of our career we are at. It helps us reflect on those who influenced us. Ultimately, *Communicable* reminds us that it is never too late as an individual to adjust and inject more of those features from those whom you have admired and regard highly today.

DALE FISHER, FRACP
Group Chief of Medicine, National University Health System
Professor, Yong Loo Lin School of Medicine,
National University of Singapore

* * *

This book was a treat to read. Nicholas Ngiam and Gabriel Yan have not only documented the pioneering work of David Allen for infectious diseases (ID) and the history of the discipline's development in Singapore, but also captured his motivations, thoughts, principles and hopes. This will benefit generations of future ID doctors and physicians in general, regardless of where they practice, and also anyone who has an interest in microbes and their impact on society. I don't think that all the multifaceted layers of David have been completely 'peeled', but Nicholas and Gabriel have almost certainly done excellently, for what can be contained in a volume like this. Readers will feel like they were sitting on a couch having a front-seat conversation with David and the authors, reviewing the people, times, and events that have and will shape the development of the specialty of Infectious Diseases not just in Singapore but beyond, and also be compelled to look within themselves to examine the 'whys' of the vocation to which they are called.

SHAWN VASOO, MBBS, MRCP, FRCPath, D (ABIM) (IM, ID),
D (ABP) (MM), FAMS
Clinical Director and Senior Consultant,
National Centre for Infectious Diseases

* * *

Want to be an icon? Read the interview Nicholas and Gabriel conducted with David Allen – and discover how David Allen attained this status. Along the way, get regaled on delicious details of the winding road ID has taken, from the days of old, to its stature as an established specialty in Singapore.

TAN BAN HOCK, MBBS, FRCP
Senior Consultant, Department of Infectious Diseases,
Singapore General Hospital
Clinical Professor, Duke-NUS Medical School

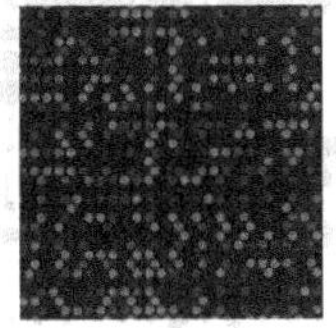

FOREWORD

A few months ago, I was in a meeting with a couple of senior doctors and a number of young trainees and MOPEX (Medical Officer Posting Exercise) MOs (Medical Officers). The junior doctors were going over the familiar litany of issues — very long hours, being overwhelmed by administrative work, not getting a chance to do direct patient care because of the demands of the electronic medical record, lack of support in dealing with patients who were aggressive because of dementia or mental health issues, bullying by seniors, etc. A senior surgeon present looked benignly round the room and began telling what I have called "old people stories" that I am unfortunately also guilty of repeating... He began by talking about how good the young people have it today, how he had to do everything himself without nurses to take blood or set [intravenous] drips, how he had to clerk thirty surgical patients in a night covering the whole of Toa Payoh Hospital (which no longer exists, having transformed into Changi General Hospital some time ago). He had to do three or four appendectomies every night and got no sleep at all nor had the chance to go "post-call". Looking around the room at the non-impressed junior doctors, he also admitted that times had been different then. He said that consent-taking [for procedures] then consisted mainly of getting someone to put their thumb on a piece of paper rather than spending half an hour explaining all the possible complications of the surgery and also all the complications of not operating. One of the juniors piped up "And (then) have to explain it all over again to a son or daughter who shows up an hour later!" Now we finally had some communication going between the young and the old — the details are different but the challenges no less real today than they had been decades ago.

When I first picked up this book written by Gabriel and Nicholas some time ago, I found myself dreading finding another collection of "old people stories" although I looked forward to some spicy morsels about some of the Infectious Diseases icons of today during their trainee days. I was pleasantly surprised to find that this book is nothing at all like that. Although it does carry on in the loose tradition of telling the story of some "Venerable, White, Senior Professor" in David's own words who had come here from Texas to blaze a trail in a new specialty in the lineage that goes as far back as Sir Gordon Arthur Ransome (and postgraduate Medicine and Neurology) or even Sir Ronald Ross (and Parasitology from 100 years ago), this book is very much a conversation between young and old practitioners of the art with insights drawn out of a unique individual who has made a lasting contribution to the clinical practice of Infectious Diseases in Singapore for the last thirty years or so.

David's uniqueness is remarkable as he still continues to do what he did thirty years ago, round on patients, walk the house-staff and trainees through the differential diagnoses and challenge their management plans. This is at a time when many if not most "expat" senior professors are expected instead to chalk up high impact publications or to score prominent appointments to add to the reputation scores that go into the rankings of the local universities rather than spend time at patients' bedsides with trainees.

This was the reason I lobbied to bring David back to Singapore as Courage Fund Visiting Professor as more than one NUH trainee in their exit assessments had commented on how great the didactic teaching/ conferences, research opportunities and infrastructure support were but the missing element was having a senior Infectious Diseases physician sit down at the bedside and spend time going over each consult in detail with them. That is where David excels, not imposing his views but forcing the trainees to justify their recommendations and occasionally provoking them with some quirky question or two. He has done that and more in the years since and has been a valuable mentor and friend to many. I am pleased that the authors decided to reproduce the recommendation letter that David wrote for me 32 years ago that did not get me into Rush Presbyterian, one of the top institutions in Chicago and the United States, but at least helped me secure a place at an inner-city community hospital not too far away that was my entry point to the US postgraduate medical education system. Reading between the lines of that letter, you will realise that David only knew me as this young ambitious MO who had referred a couple of Prof Tan Yew Oo's oncology patients to him but he still managed to fill two pages for a decent recommendation!

This book is full of interesting anecdotes and perspectives on stories which have been told before but this time from the point of view of two very literate young ID/Microbiology doctors, one of whom has aspirations to being a Chinese literary scholar judging from the aphorisms colouring the text. The final chapter of the book is perhaps the most interesting as it looks to the future, to the world so many of us are facing and not just the senior surgeon trying to engage stressed out junior doctors. Frankly, I am glad that I am not an MO in 2024 as the future is a lot more uncertain today than it was in 1992, when finishing Advanced Specialty Training (Advanced Specialty Training) would almost certainly mean a relatively comfortable life and a clear pathway either to private practice or to a rewarding senior public sector career. The frank discussions and insightful ideas raised in this conversation give us all hope that we will find a way. Even if there are no simple answers, the story is told in such an engaging way that my wife, who picked up the book from our coffee table a couple of weeks ago, could not put it down! Enjoy!

Paul Ananth Tambyah
Professor of Medicine
Senior Consultant
Infectious Diseases Physician

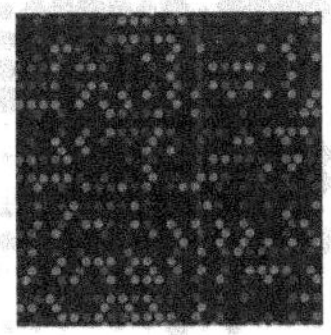

PREFACE

I first met David Allen when I was a medical officer. It was the peak of the COVID-19 pandemic, and the hospital wards were bursting with patients. Having to round a long inpatient list with a highly prolific senior consultant felt like a potentially daunting task. However, any anxiety that I had initially felt about the morning rounds were immediately put to ease by his candour and easy-going demeanour. His first words to me — *"Don't apologise, I am here to be at your service."*

Over the week, what struck me was that despite his incredible wealth of knowledge and experience, he was always able to meet junior doctors at their level. He would always listen. He would be quick to engage my input on managing patients in a collaborative fashion. He encouraged me to think, to voice my opinions, and to advocate for the patients I was seeing. He inspired me to want to constantly be better as a physician, and to do the best for the patient in front of us.

My experience was not a unique one. David has been an inspiration to so many others, in his decades-long career. Thus, we have sought to encapsulate this narrative of resilience, intellect, and compassion — a story that unfolds against the backdrop of the ever-evolving landscape of Infectious Diseases in Singapore. In his career, David has devoted himself to improving the systems and processes that he has been a part of, and to also continually impart knowledge and the right values to the next generation of physicians. The chapters of this book trace his remarkable journey through his lens and voice: as a distinguished physician who came from afar, chronicling his immeasurable impact on Infectious Diseases as a specialty in Singapore, as well as on a personal level, his impact on the lives of numerous young doctors who have walked the corridors of Singapore's public hospitals.

It is our hope that by immortalizing his words and experiences in this text, David's life and work will continue to be a positive influence for countless future generations to come.

Nicholas Ngiam
July 2024

I first heard about David Allen when I was in my first year of training in Infectious Diseases, at the National University Hospital. I vividly recall Alvin Wang, then my senior in training, telling me that the Father of Infectious Diseases in Singapore was covering the wards, and that it would be a good opportunity to tag along and learn from him. He was a walking encyclopaedia of infectious diseases knowledge, but there was a caveat — *'his ward rounds can be very long'*. I was intrigued. Back then, I did not yet appreciate the history of my specialty. It had dealt with conditions that have plagued humans since time immemorial, but what was surprising to me was that I could still be within more than touching distance with its founder. At least our local one. I was, unfortunately, unable to attend his ward rounds, a rookie barely able to keep his head above the water. I will also admit, frankly, that long ward rounds have never been particularly enticing.

I was to meet him in the flesh during my final year of training. I was invited for lunch, once again by Alvin, during my rotation at Ng Teng Fong General Hospital. Undoubtedly, I was a tad anxious. He was, after all, this White, senior professor from the States, and there is always a palpable fear of appearing unintelligible. We veered away from the topic of Infectious Diseases, and ended up discussing about the States instead — about people's rights, guns, and the then President of the United States, Donald Trump. It was also when I first heard him intone about his near brush with death, when he stared down the barrel of a gun (which we got him to recount in Chapter 1). He was congenial and gregarious, and I have been at ease ever since.

Later on that year, I did eventually have consults with him one afternoon. It didn't feel long. In fact, there was plenty to absorb, and it was too short a time for that. Crucially, it was during this event that he conveyed a message that has stuck with me ever since. I was managing a particularly difficult case, and was feeling hesitant about the next step. I was also about to take my Infectious Diseases exit examinations. Uncertainty was not supposed to be in the vocabulary. He saw me agonizing, and recognised its importance.

"Throughout your career, in the management of your patients, it is always important to remain uncomfortable."

I understood then the profoundness of his words. He affirmed that I had done my duty of care for my patient, whilst reassuring me that I did not have to know, in fact, did not have the *right* to know, everything under the sun to have done so. He also set, there and then, the minimum expectation to abide by for the rest of my career — that I remain uncomfortable for each and every patient I was to encounter. I still try to do so.

'Communicable' is about a conversation with David Allen. It is, in essence, taking a history from Infectious Diseases, the specialty. The history of David Allen; the history of infectious diseases and Infectious Diseases, the specialty; the history of Singapore and the specialty in Singapore. It is an ode to heroes in the field, past and present — David will be the first to acknowledge that he has built Infectious Diseases in Singapore on the foundations laid by others. It is these others, our pioneers, that we hope to illuminate and remember as well within the pages of this book. *'Communicable'* is also about the future. The future that collided with the present in the form of a pandemic, a future that is potentially fraught with even more perils than the one just past. The late Dr Paul Farmer, an Infectious Diseases physician and public health champion, once said, *'Epidemics, like war, are seen to crash down upon us from a cloudless sky in part because we aren't attentive to storms of our own making.'* We aim to forecast some of these storms in our consultations with David, and

what we could do to mitigate the devastation, if not prevent them. Finally, '*Communicable*' is also about being a doctor. It is about what it means to have a long and fulfilling career. It is about tempering expectations, yet at the same time attaining lofty ideals. It is about mastering the art and science of Medicine. It is about reminding ourselves of the privilege we have been tasked with — to serve the vulnerable.

'*All trainees deserve to be guided by physicians who see in them the possibility of making medicine better.*' These are the words of Dr Lisa Rosenbaum, an Assistant Professor of Medicine at Harvard Medical School. It encapsulates perfectly what David has done for us. '*Communicable*' is thus about sharing David with people who have met him, and with those who may yet do. I hope his words inspire you as much as they have for me. May they make you comfortably uncomfortable.

Gabriel Yan
July 2024

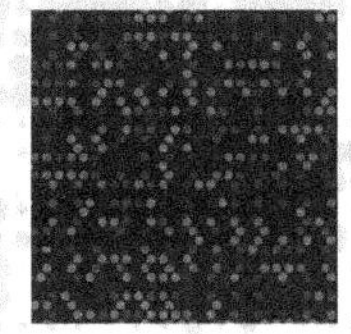

PROLOGUE

—

ars longa, vita brevis
'skilfulness takes time and life is short'

We start off, like most gatherings in Singapore, with a meal. It's nearly noon, on the day of the first Saturday screening of '*Oppenheimer*' and '*Barbie*' (*circa* 2023). We are seated in a cosy cafe that served Thai food, which was unintentionally chosen in preparation for the afternoon's marathon dialogue. David is running a few minutes late, but only because the venue is situated at an obscure location in the building. He arrives, unhurried, and we order our food. He is, of course, no stranger to Thai cuisine. He also laments that he's lost the popular vote for his group movie outing later — the lots had been cast for '*Barbie*'. We jest that he might need something light-hearted after a heavy-going session. The food arrives and he loads up on the *chilli padi* (bird's eye chilli). And then he throws a curveball.

"What are we doing again today, fellas?"

His eyebrows are furrowed. The tone is more serious than his usual avuncular demeanour. Hadn't we been through this with him before? This meeting had not been arranged on the spur of the moment. We had been planning this for some time, and he had agreed to participate right from the beginning. We had even met up prior, to go through some of the ideas, and the questions had been prepared, sent, and approved. The dates in our calendars had been blocked since a few months back. But this was his style of doing things. He knew what he was doing, but he wanted to be sure that *we* knew what we were doing. He was adopting his usual consultancy and advisory role that we typically experienced when we went on rounds with him in the hospital.

We elaborate again. He was a bit of an enigma to many of us junior doctors. He was the person we sought when we ran into diagnostic or management dilemmas for our patients, and he always had a quote-worthy anecdote ready in his pocket to share with us, like a piece of gum. And it typically stuck. But beyond all that, we had no idea who David Michael Allen was. We were upfront and laid our cards on the table. We wanted to be historians, to document, for posterity, the history of our specialty and its founding father in Singapore. We wanted this to be about personal development, to leverage on his own experiences garnered over the decades as he journeyed from being a junior doctor to a senior consultant. And we wanted to engage in a bit of forecasting, peering into his thoughts so that we could predict the future, or at least better anticipate what's potentially coming our way. He understands all this, and is seemingly reassured. And then he fires another warning shot.

"You know, a group from NUS[1] has asked me before, too. They wanted to interview me and write my story down, but I'd declined it back then."

Was he getting cold feet? That wasn't quite like him. The rationale behind his rebuff was much more fundamental. It was down to the fact that he felt that he would have been sharing it with the wrong audience. His story was personal, thus it had to be meaningful, and for it to be meaningful, it had to be shared with the people he knew. In telling us this little backstory, he was letting us know that he had gifted us this privilege. Not that we didn't already know we were treading on hallowed ground, but it was a reminder to us that we were fortunate to have this opportunity arise. He sees that we understand, and makes one final, specific request, laying down the rules of engagement.

"I want you to go *mano a mano*. I don't want you pulling your punches."

He didn't want this interview to be filled with the typical reverence and awe experienced by junior doctors when they encountered him. This was a particular bugbear of his, to have his word treated as gospel truth. He had been experiencing this since he had first set foot on our shores — the Asian culture of deference to elders and superiors. It was different to what he had been brought up with, and it was a losing battle he had long fought against. He wanted his students to question doctrine, to push against boundaries, to topple long-held beliefs. He liked to be challenged, and he was invigorated by it. And if he was proven wrong, he'd be even more delighted to know that his students had surpassed their master. It was clear though that it wasn't going to be a fair fight. He was, after all, venerable, White, and on top of all that, a senior professor from the States.[2] He's satisfied to proceed now, and with lunch concluded, we adjourn back to our hunting ground — the National University Hospital (NUH) — for the afternoon's activity.

We settle down, him separated from us across a six-foot-long meeting table. It's almost like a job interview, and even though we were going to be the ones interrogating, it was clear who would be running the show. Hopefully, our lunchtime conversation wouldn't turn out to be the precursor of the Abilene paradox.[3] And after doing some sound checks, we begin.

For throwing us a little off balance earlier on during lunch, we thought we'd catch him a little off guard with a question not included in our agreed-upon list. Not that it would have fazed him. You can learn a lot about a person by what they read, and by what they recommend, and we start off by asking David to come up with a few titles that inspired him, and that could inspire the next generation.

"There is no perfect book for everyone. One should read any book that stimulates your mind, to give you a perspective on the world. For example, '*The Winds of War*', '*The Moviegoer*', '*As I Lay Dying*'. Classic books that delve into the human experience. What it is like to live, to love, to suffer, and to be mortal." These were all works of fiction. There were no inspiring biographies of Infectious Diseases[4] folk heroes such as Paul Farmer in '*Mountains Beyond Mountains*', or buccaneering adventures of viral hunters such as Peter Piot in '*No Time to Lose*'. There were no epic histories of Medicine such as Roy Porter's '*The Greatest Benefit to Mankind*' or ID canon such as Randy Shilts' journalistic interrogation of the HIV[5] epidemic in '*And the Band Played On*'. A quote from a more contemporary American author, George R. R. Martin, summarises his choices succinctly — '*A reader lives a thousand lives before he dies. The man who never reads lives only one.*'

He elaborates further. "I think we are reminded daily as Infectious Diseases physicians — we may not always allow ourselves to step back and look at it — that we deal with important questions every day that human beings confront. Example: life, quality of life, length of life, meaning of life, value of life. We deal with them in a somewhat mechanistic and algorithmic way. Our patients are not widgets, they are not items. They are human beings and they have emotions and feelings and context and values that we may not always understand. You can become human through other ways, through exploring the arts, and literature and music. There are lots of ways to be human." The practice of Medicine, to him, was an art, a humanity. You can get all the science from the textbooks and journal articles, but it was not going to tell you how to be a doctor. To quote an eminent Canadian physician from the 19th century, Dr William Osler — '*The good physician treats the disease; the great physician treats the patient who has the disease.*'

He concludes. "By immersing ourselves in the bigger world, outside of the pure sciences of Infectious Diseases, we allow ourselves to be human."

We've barely begun, and here, he gives us our first piece of gum to chew. And it stuck. We were in for a treat.

Notes

[1] National University of Singapore

[2] This is a caricature of himself that David frequently likes to bring up to trainees. We wouldn't have the temerity to label him as such.

[3] The Abilene paradox was coined by Jerry Harvey, a management expert, following a disastrous family outing to Abilene, Texas, for dinner, 50 miles away from where they were residing. Everyone had initially agreed that it was a great idea to undertake, but it eventually turned out that no one really wanted to make the arduous journey in the first place, and were only going along with the perceived flow.[6] The paradox describes collective fallacy, a group dynamic in which everyone agrees to an action plan that none of the individual members actually wanted to partake in.

[4] Throughout the book, the terminology 'Infectious Diseases', with the initial capitalization of the first alphabets of each word, or 'ID' for short, is used to describe the medical specialty which manages patients with conditions caused by pathogens. When used as 'infectious diseases', without the initial capitalization of the first alphabets, it represents the diseases caused by pathogens.

[5] Human immunodeficiency virus

[6] Jerry B. Harvey, 'The Abilene paradox: The management of agreement', *Organizational Dynamics*, 1974;3(1):63–80.

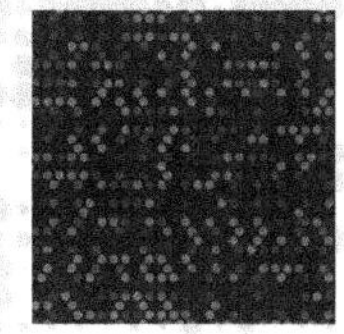

CONTENTS

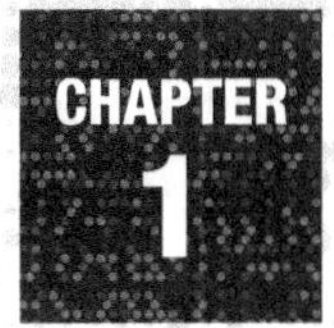

ORIGINS

—

sic parvis magna
'greatness from small beginnings'

There have been many paternal figures throughout the history of Medicine. Hippocrates, the Father of Medicine, elevated the practice of Medicine by infusing intellectual rigour, disaffiliating it from supernatural and religious healing. Dr William Osler, the Father of modern Medicine, transformed the profession into an art, being the exemplar of an astute diagnostician with impeccable bedside manners. He reformed the medical education system as well by establishing the first formal residency programme for doctors. The particular fields of Microbiology and Infectious Diseases are not devoid of luminaries as well. Antonie van Leeuwenhoek, the Father of Microbiology, crafted the first microscopes with the capability to observe microorganisms, which he then termed 'animalcules'. This opened up a previously unexplored dimension of understanding diseases, resulting in the replacement of the miasmatic theory, where the spread of diseases was believed to be due to bad air, with that of the germ theory, where infections by microorganisms were the direct causation of certain conditions. Dr Robert Koch, the Father of modern Bacteriology, developed the techniques to culture bacteria in laboratories, and in so doing, discovered the causative agents of anthrax (*Bacillus anthracis*) and tuberculosis (*Mycobacterium tuberculosis*). He is synonymous with Koch's postulates, which currently still governs the principles of determining causality between a pathogen and a disease.

Dr John Snow, the Father of modern Epidemiology, did investigative work on a mid-19th century cholera outbreak in London that led him to conclude that a contaminated public water pump, at Broad Street, was the source of the epidemic. The contagion subsequently ceased with the removal of its pump handle. Dr Ignaz Semmelweis, the Father of Infection Control, noticed a difference in puerperal fever mortality rates between two maternity clinics, with higher rates in the one staffed by medical students compared to that staffed by midwives. He discerned the culprits to be medical students, who went straight from performing cadaveric autopsies to examining pregnant mothers without washing their hands. A simple fix by instituting hand hygiene (handwashing) prior to physical examination of the mothers resulted in plummeting mortality rates.

Yet, to be the founding father of a new paradigm in Medicine may have many different meanings. All of the greats mentioned above brought about a significant change in practice. They made a breakthrough and instituted changes which significantly altered the path which Medicine took. They made the art and science of Medicine better. They were the pioneers in their nascent fields. Regrettably, for some, the novelty of their findings, despite their potential for immense impact, did not take root immediately. The discoveries by Drs John Snow and Ignaz Semmelweis were politically sensitive, and also conflicted with the miasmatic theory held by the medical establishment during their time. Widespread recognition for their work only came about posthumously. They did not attain a following, which some of the others did. Hippocrates and Dr William Osler both achieved cult-like status during their lifetimes, and not unlike biological fathers, had 'progenies' which propagated their thoughts and practices.

Our lens now shifts into focus: we examine David Michael Allen, the Father of Infectious Diseases in Singapore. The reason he has been conferred this honour is keenly obvious to us. We, the interviewers, are descendants, and the fruits of his labour. In simplistic terms, he established a new branch of Medicine here in Singapore, the specialty to which we belong — Infectious Diseases. He brought about an ideology to the medical profession in Singapore that first became pervasive and then subsequently, a necessity. Before he arrived on our shores, Infectious Diseases as a specialty did not exist. It may have seemed irrelevant back then, since a substantial amount of medical practice in that era involved some manner of infectious diseases. And it may still seem so even now. But he brought gravitas, professionalism and, more importantly, relevance, to the subject matter. And it would also be an irrelevant discussion to wonder if there could have been some other to have made a similar impact. The fact of the matter is that he succeeded first. And he continues to have an influence in the Infectious Diseases realm here in Singapore. But more profoundly, he continues to guide the next generation of doctors, not just those in our specialty. Speak to any medical professional, from students to emeritus professors, who have crossed paths with him, and they never fail to come away enlightened.

There is a Chinese idiom, '光前裕后', [guāng qián yù hòu], which means *'bringing honour to one's ancestors reaps benefits for future generations'*. And that's why we are here. We wanted to understand more about him. How had he become the person he was? Why did he come? Where was he headed next? What else did he have for us? We had learnt, and still had much to learn, from him, and we thought it selfish if it could not be shared for posterity. And thus, we begin where all stories should begin — his origins. How did David Allen come to be?

"My father, Abraham Allen, was the child of immigrants from Lithuania and Russia. They did not speak much English. Very little. He grew up speaking Yiddish and English in an immigrant community which consisted of East Europeans, Irish and Puerto Ricans. So, very poor, and lots of fisticuffs. My father's family ended up in what's called Bayonne, New Jersey, which was an immigrant community near Ellis Island, a central place where many immigrants in the early 1900s came through."

Ellis Island is situated just adjacent to the Statue of Liberty, in New York City. Around the turn of the 20th century, immigrants from the Old World seeking their fortunes in the new one would traverse the Atlantic and enter the United States through New York Harbour. After an arduous, sea-sickening journey, they were typically uplifted by the sight of Lady Liberty glistening in the sun, shortly before docking at Ellis Island to be processed by immigration authorities.

"And my mother, Sariet Allen, was also the grandchild of East European immigrants. Her grandparents were from Ukraine and Russia, but her parents had been born in the United States. My mother's family had come through Galveston, Texas, and then migrated to Louisiana and Mississippi in the southern United States where they settled. The East Europeans settled in the small communities in the southern United States. The people that came through Ellis Island settled mostly in the northeast into enclaves."

David is an Ashkenazi Jew — a descendant of Jews who live or once lived in Central or Eastern Europe. The mass migration of the Jews to America in the early 1900s was precipitated by rising anti-Semitism in Eastern Europe. At that point in time, only the Jews in North America and Western Europe were emancipated, and America was seen as an ideal destination. Ideal for its relative dearth of threats and abundance of opportunities. This insight into his family background explains a little with regards to David's psyche — the rebel who doesn't always look to conform, the vagabond who's never truly settled in one place. Not at least until now.

One also can't help but notice the parallels between his background and those of ours. More of a pull rather than a push factor, our forefathers left the coastal southern provinces of China, from Guangzhou and Fujian, to seek better job prospects under the British here in Singapore. This, though, occurred nearly a century before David's ancestors made the move across the Atlantic.

David presses on. "My father came back from the Korean conflict [Korean War, 1950–1953] and he had been accepted into Rutgers University. But because of all the military guys coming out, there was a year waiting list, and he and his family had no money. He used the G.I. Bill and was accepted in the University of Oklahoma. My parents met in the University of Oklahoma and then settled in a small town in West Texas called Abilene. When he got there, it was probably 30,000 people. When I was there, it was maybe 60- to 70,000 people. And it's a sort of a town of commerce, in the sense. There's a lot of cotton, sorghum and cattle with a little bit of oil. It was kind of a convergence of those things in a small, little town."

Sorghum?

"Sorghum is a grain. It's used in feed for animals. So, cattle and pigs and stuff."

He continues painting the landscape of the pastoral setting of his hometown and the humble journey of his father's. "So that's what it was. It was primarily agricultural and some commerce, small businesses. And the only reason he went there — there's no East Europeans there — was because he had no money. And they offered him a job at, I think, $55 a month when he graduated from University of Oklahoma with a pharmacy degree. He took it because his parents had nothing."

Although it wasn't as pastoral as he had initially made it out to be. "And the town also had a military base. It was a strategic military base because it had an airplane called a B-52, which is a long-range bomber, that stayed in the air 24-hours a day. It would circle about a 150-kilometre circumference, and it had launch codes for the intercontinental ballistic missiles. And there were missile silos outside my town that were buried underground. The reason that plane was in the air 24-hours a day was in case that Russia bombed Central Command, that were war to have taken place, the US military could still launch from the plane."

"I grew up going to primary and middle school and high school, inculcated in what to do when a nuclear bomb goes off. We would hide under our desks because that would save us from the blast, or we would hide in the hall with our heads down. I grew up with that. That was pretty cool."

This would have been at the height of the Cold War, around the period of the Cuban Missile Crisis when the world teetered on the edge of an all-out nuclear war between the United States and the Soviet Union. One isn't too sure if it had been truly comprehensible to him, back then, the impact should there have been a nuclear incident in the vicinity. Most buildings would be obliterated within a 300-metre radius; most living beings would be annihilated from the radiation within a 1-kilometre radius; and third-degree burns would be suffered universally up to a radius of 2 kilometres from the blast epicentre. He was, in all likelihood, just playing it cool, leveraging on his old bragging rights from childhood. He notices how unnerved we were and reels us back in, to less apocalyptic memories. "But it was a town with a lot of outdoors, so I spent a lot of my youth outside — hunting, fishing, camping, hiking, chasing, playing."

More importantly, he was also a bibliophile, and he credits his parents for nurturing this. "My mother and father read enormously. My father read a book every couple of days, and they were quality literature. My mother read everything from comic books to high literature to whatever. She was not discriminating. That influenced me, seeing them read. I read encyclopaedias, and lots of biographies and fiction. I read trash fiction as well as more classical literature. I read a lot."

There were books, and then there was jazz. David enjoyed jazz. "My father played classical music in the house from a record. And jazz." He reflected on his prior musical aspirations, recalling his childhood idol. "I had a saxophone for a while. I wanted to be like Coltrane. The saxophone didn't work out." With that, he lets loose the jazz aficionado in one of the authors (Gabriel). One of the most influential American jazz artists of the 20th century, John Coltrane regularly sought to break musical boundaries in his short lifetime. He was also a heroin addict, burning his candle at both ends before finally succumbing to liver cancer at the tender age of 40. Musical idols of that era were supposed to include mainstream names such as Elvis or the Beatles. But anyone who hero-worships Coltrane deserves his place in another category altogether. The next statement cemented it definitively. "And I did take care of Miles Davis. He was wasting away. But he's a genius." Miles Davis, American jazz trumpeter and bandleader, another unfettered, epoch-maker in the jazz universe. Rumours had always been rife that Miles had AIDS[1] and was on AZT,[2] and that he had died of complications associated with the former. David bites his tongue, neither denying nor confirming the rumour.

He doesn't give us time to dwell on these fanboy moments, but instead, clinically dissects the reasoning behind their brilliance. Like a true diagnostician. It's as if we had sidetracked him from his true love, Medicine. "Many of them had substance abuse issues. And it was part of the life. But they [the substance abuse] didn't detract from their artistry. It probably added, honestly." It is a bit of a taboo to even talk about chewing gum in Singapore, let alone waxing-lyrical about drugs and substance abuse. Having digressed momentarily, we return back to his growing up years, and he briefly mentions his siblings. He was the youngest of three. "My brothers, Steven and Ira Allen, are five years and three years older than me. Seeing what they were up to influenced me — good and bad. One's a physician, one is an IT guy and an inventor with IBM."

He goes on to talk about his childhood education. "My school, and my community, was very religious. I am not of the religion that was dominant there. I was the only person of my religion throughout my schooling in that community. My friend's parents knew that I was of different ethnicity and religion and didn't like it." Regrettably, the fact that racism is a product of nurture rather than nature sticks out here. "But my friends could not care less. We friends are all the same. We're all dirty and whatever. I was influenced by them because they're a product of their culture. I would go hang out at their houses and see how they lived differently, what their parents valued, which was sometimes different than what our family did. All that influenced me. It helped me to assimilate into the new culture; to not learn the language of my ancestors, Yiddish; to question the rituals of my heritage; to try not to be 'other'. I was, and am, never embarrassed by my heritage and religion. Just that, as a young person in particular, I didn't want that to be my sole redeeming features."

Formal education appears, at least to us, to have been a rite of passage for the children in his community, and not a ticket to success. Or perhaps success was measured by a different yardstick in his community. "The educational system there was really not structured for higher learning. It wasn't a classic education. We could read and write. I went to an elite university because I did well for all of my exams. But most of the rest couldn't. Maybe 20% of us went to university." Despite the cultural norms at that time, he did not conform to expectation but instead pursued higher education.

"I went to counselling for what to do at the end of secondary school, or high school, in the States. I told my counsellor that I was going to university. And they told me not to, that that was a waste of time. Religion had nothing to do with it. *'University will fill your head with silly ideas that are of no use to anyone. We need tradesmen and air conditioning repairmen now. I can get you into a trade school. You'll be a value to the community and make a contribution. Instead, if you go to university, you'll be a waste of resources and time.'* That was the general feeling — that the higher education was not of value to the community."

One's cultural background definitely plays an important role in influencing major life's decisions. Here we see again, how critical his family values were in his formative years. The seeds of *his* love for education, to nurture and mentor others, had been sown since his youth. "I just happened to have a family which values education. My heritage aligns very much with the values of Asian communities. Family, education — these were most important. And at the time, it didn't matter how you got educated or what you were educated in. You could be a historian, you could be an English major, you could be a doctor. They were all of equal value. Education was the value. To be an educated person was considered a virtue, whatever you were educated in. And not necessarily to be a professional. My mother didn't hound me to be a doctor. This message may be different from what Singaporean children hear. It was more like, '*You will be the pride of the family and your brothers if you get educated. We don't care what you do.*'"

Asian and Jewish families undoubtedly resemble one another in terms of the emphasis placed on education, although the rationale behind it may have some subtle differences. Asian families, in particular Chinese families, have a distinct stereotype — the value of higher education is a means to a well-paying job. Children in Asian families are typically pressured by their parents, unwittingly or not, to strive to be in professions such as doctors or lawyers. It was a matter of status, a matter of financial security. In Singapore, parents care a lot about what you do. It might be cliché, but he wasn't too far off from hitting the nail on its head.

As a matter of trivia, an origin story from the United States would not be complete without guns. The Second Amendment of the US Constitution lawfully bestows upon its citizens the right to bear arms, although it has become a bone of contention in recent decades. Hailing from Texas, the foremost state in the US with the highest number of registered weapons, David contributed to that statistic. We probed him a little more about his own gun-toting habits.

"My first gun was a BB gun when I was eleven or twelve. And then I got a small calibre rifle when I was fourteen. I got my first shotgun when I was fourteen or sixteen. And the .22, which is a small calibre rifle, was used to hunt rabbits when we went camping. My friends and I would then skin and eat them, though we didn't need it for food. And the shotgun was used for dove and quail hunting, and we would eat them as well. I mean, that was kind of fun, to grill them and barbecue." It comes across as a bit blasé to us, but only because of our background. Military conscription is required of all able-bodied males in Singapore, typically at the age of 18. We were each handed our 'wife', or what our rifles are otherwise known as, on the first day of enlistment. And for many of us, it was very much a heavy burden rather than a new toy — it was physically and metaphorically an anchor around our neck; cleaning inspections were a chore with impossible standards to achieve; every single bullet or empty shell had to be accounted for; and any missing part of the rifle could potentially lead to punitive outcomes for the soldier. It was not fun.

He knows where this topic is headed towards — gun violence in the States — and he continued to share light-hearted anecdotes. "Your buddy would be maybe fifty to a hundred metres away from you, when a shotgun's pellets' velocity has dropped off. Maybe your buddy would shoot you every once in a while, just to give you a little sting of the pellets, but not in malice. So, yeah, I grew up in a gun culture, but not the gun culture that exists now. People didn't have cannons [semi-automatic weapons] in their pockets, and I can't recall shootings like there exists now. There were no school shootings then, but we did have stabbings. My community had a lot of young men violence, in the '70s. There was a lot of cultural turmoil from the '60s, from the Vietnam conflict, and so, there were gang fights and stabbings in the school."

Despite the absence of guns in schools, it still didn't seem to have been a particularly safe environment to have grown up in. He recounts what had been done in his community to dissipate the violence. "One of the things they did was that they opened up all the sports facilities. It used to be you had to pay a dollar or two to go play basketball on weekends or something to rent the court. But they wanted all the young men's energy expended so they opened all these things up. Idle bodies and minds were occupied, and energies depleted. There was less enthusiasm for violence once they were worn out from sports."

Not infrequently, David has enthralled each batch of ID trainees during his ward rounds with anecdotes about how he had been shot at, but thankfully survived. We got him to give us a blow-by-blow account of the incident for us again, for posterity.

"When 16, I was out with four other close friends. Around 9 pm, we went to a teenager hangout in Abilene, which was a pool hall where we could meet other friends, boast, brag, tell lies, play pool, drink beer…" He pauses momentarily before interjecting himself. "Although underage."

He carries on with his escapades. "Listen to loud rock and roll from a juke box, flirt and mingle." His portrayal of himself seemed almost unrecognisable to us. This was David from a different chapter of his life. "The crowd was generally between 16–18 years old. There were always a few older boys, aged 19–21 years, or men, from the local military base present as well. The air base was 10–15 miles from town, and it was a world that interacted very little with the town — except for the drone of the B-52s. The town liked the airmen to spend their pay checks in town and then leave. These young airmen were not from the area, and often not from Texas. They were from a different culture at that time, and away from their families, girlfriends and support structures. They were generally bored on the airbase when not on duty, and were seeking a bit of entertainment and female companionship. The US military was essentially all male then."

After setting the scene, he jumps right into the action. "One young, possibly 20-year-old, airman was awkwardly flirting with our female friend, and she was annoyed. She was not my girlfriend. He wouldn't stop. I told him his flirting skills were wanting, though not exactly in those words, and that he should stop. He was not pleased. It exacerbated his frustration and embarrassment, being told this by a 16-year-old. He was a bit inebriated. I was not. He said, '*Let's take this outside.*'" This was all bravado. David was being challenged to a fight, and he was not one to back down easily.

"He was alone, and I was with my four friends. It was understood that the issue was between the airman and myself. My friends were witnesses, 'seconds' in the duelling era, not active participants. On stepping outside, the airman opined, '*This place is too crowded, let's do this at site X,*' indicating a quiet neighbourhood nearby. I agreed."

The narrative takes a turn similar to a cinematic action film. "He drove there alone. I was in a car with my buddies, and the verbal equivalent of a Māori haka took place in the car amongst my friends to prepare me.

On arrival, the street was quiet. The nearby homes had porch lights on, streetlights were present but not bright, and they were augmented by the two cars' cabin lighting. But it was otherwise dark. The cars disgorged their contents, and he and I faced each other and took our stances, ready to strike." You can almost hear the legendary Ennio Morricone's epic soundtrack from Sergio Leone's Western, '*The Good, the Bad, and the Ugly*', simmering in the background.

"He almost immediately said, '*Let me take my shirt off as I don't want to get your blood on it when I hit you,*' and walked to the boot of his car while taking his shirt off. I smirked and said, '*Whatever*'. He opened the boot, bent over and put his shirt in the boot, and stood up holding a rifle, now aimed at me from about 12–15 metres away." You can sense the blood immediately draining from his and his friends' faces. Adrenaline kicks in and the impulse for flight overwhelms the response to fight.

"I bolted to my left toward the front yard and sparse trees of the nearest home. My friends literally scattered. All of us ran in different directions, some taking diversionary tactics. Shots rang out within 2–3 seconds of my initial movements and hit a car parked on the street in front me, before I could get to the trees. Sparse though they were, they would help. Then a shot hit a tree in front of me, and then the street pavement to my left. One of my friends was likely an easier target. A total of 6 shots were fired. Then we heard a car door close, wheels squeal, and he was gone. One friend had pulled a weather door off a nearby home trying to get in. We initially couldn't find another friend — he dove under our car when the shooting started and stayed until he was sure the coast was clear. I had made it about 500 metres down the street, bobbing and weaving amongst the trees in the front yards of the homes on the street. There were no front yard fences in that community. No one had been hit." It was not the first time he had narrated the story to us, but the tone of it varies each time. Today, he's convivial and relates the incident to us somewhat blithely. There had been times previously where it had been no laughing matter. The intention behind the sharing is clear to us. It had been a fortuitous escape for him and his friends, and it must still have affected him somewhat. Behind every scar is an untold story of survival. This was his brush with death, his invisible scar.

He concludes this subtopic on a more serious note — his thoughts on the Second Amendment and the right to bear arms. He thoroughly understands the underlying rationale behind the ratification of this amendment, and seeks to clarify it for us. "As a young person, guns were for hunting, both for food and recreation, sporting, for target practice and skeet shooting, and to a lesser degree, protection from coyotes and mountain lions who kill your livestock, from vipers when camping or hiking, and from people intending to harm you. Owning a gun in West Texas at that time wasn't considered macho, but an essential tool for those living in rural areas. Fewer urbanites had guns."

"The US Second Amendment granting the right to keep and bear arms was derived from English common law. Its purpose in the US Constitution was, and is, to allow citizens to protect themselves and their property. Those who view the US Constitution as Originalists, as do the politically conservative majority of the current US Supreme Court, state that we are not able to contextualize the Constitution to modern circumstances, including the availability of weapons capable of rapid mass killings." The current conservative majority of the US Supreme Court, now in 2024, rigidly determine that the text of the US Constitution should be interpreted according to the era that it was formulated in. In this instance, 1791, for the Second Amendment. It is mind-boggling for us, but it is not our prerogative to comment. David himself believes that it, and any of its amendments, is a living document which should be interpreted with the times.

"Thus, there is essentially very little restriction to ownership. One can walk about with guns on display, blame mental health issues for their use in mass killings, place the burden on unsuspecting victims of shootings to protect themselves from random mass shootings, rather than restricting the circumstances in which people can have guns and the lethality of the guns they can keep." Mass shootings in US schools frequently come to the fore for their lethality and their tragedy. In schools in Singapore, children undergo fire drills. In the US, they have lockdown drills. Children should not be growing up in such an environment.

He rigorously states his stance. "The majority of Americans want more background checks and cooling off periods for people who want to buy guns. The majority of Americans want assault weapons banned. I am in favour of both." The US has been 'attempting' to curb gun violence with every gun death and mass shooting, with the Democrats seeking restrictions, but the Conservatives seeking, at least on the surface, to arm ever more citizens. The complexities of government and governance within the US have, bewilderingly, resulted in firearm sales continuing to rise year on year. We wouldn't want to appear presumptuous but to us, this was the definition of insanity — doing the same thing over and over again and expecting different results. It seems like such a simple issue that could be resolved with some common sense, but it has become much too convoluted and politicized in recent years. We sign off on this topic for now and head back to the main conversation.

For all that he has told us thus far, it was still not clear how this unconventional background led to the pursuit of a career in Medicine. In fact, the route David took was far more circuitous than one would imagine. "When I was at university [Rice University], I wanted to be an oceanographer, and I did some summer months as an intern in an Oceanography institute." In working with the oceanographers, David quickly came to certain conclusions. "I realised some of the questions that were being raised, fundamental questions of physiology being asked in animal models, were with the intent of better understanding human physiology." But these left him unfulfilled. "I thought I would rather raise them by dealing with humans directly, than with animals in the ocean."

He started having second thoughts. "Plus, the life of an oceanographer was not very attractive. Mostly, you're hustling for grants. You're not on a ship drinking wine and hanging out with chicks in bikinis. You're mostly in the lab writing grants. I did it for a couple of years and I hung out with them. They were very nice and very bright people. Capable people. And we're doing good basic science, but I wanted a little more immediacy. The nice thing about Medicine is — you see a patient, you make a change, or you do Science, and, you can see the results. Whereas we were mapping the neurons in a sea slug called *Aplysia*. It was quite interesting." This time, it's a little bit more difficult to determine if David is being sardonic. An *Aplysia* may sound interesting enough to us, but perhaps only as a Chinese delicacy. But we digress. David continues, with the characteristic twinkle in his eye, "The guys involved became very famous, but I was like, '*Better them than me.*'"

In the States, Medicine is a postgraduate degree. For his undergraduate years at Rice University, he had majored in Biology and Molecular Biology, with a minor in Anthropology. His post-graduate medical school years began thereafter in the University of Texas Southwestern Medical School. Similar to most post-graduate medical degrees, it consisted of two years of pre-clinical work followed by another two years of clinical work. "It's part of the University of Texas system, which is underwritten by the State of Texas, which was quite wealthy at the time that I was there. They trained PhDs, MD-PhDs and MDs. There have been five Nobel laureates on faculty at the time or within a few years of my matriculation. Southwestern was focused on turning out clinician scientists. That's what *they* wanted." You can sense the irony when he brings this issue up. This rebelling against the expectations of the establishment is a recurring theme throughout the interview. We saw it earlier when his high school counsellor poured scorn on his ambitions for a tertiary education, and we would come across it again when he made the move to Singapore. The apparent goals of his university, to be a clinician scientist on the path to a Nobel prize, wasn't in line with what he was envisioning his future to be. He wasn't seeking personal recognition. He just wanted to help people, in his own customary way.

David reflected with nostalgia the vast differences between medical training during his time compared with the way it was now. "As a third-year medical student, you were expected to take on a patient or two when you start your clinical rotations. You are what they call the 'sub-intern'. You work with, and in parallel to, the interns, but not really. Primarily you deal with your medical resident, or the equivalent of an MO,[3] who keeps an eye on you, to make sure you aren't causing harm. The difference between my experience as a student and current days is that I gained hands-on-experience. I started putting in lines and drawing blood, and then at the end of my third year, I was allowed to do LPs,[4] and then I delivered babies in my fourth year, performed episiotomies and closed them. You would be invited to participate in the surgical theatre, and you're essentially a human retractor. At that time, laparoscopy was not available, so you got to observe and assist in a minor way with lots of surgery. You were evaluated both on your knowledge and your capacity to work in a team as a contributing member. And a little bit on your technical skills, whether you could do some of the things that were asked — if you put in a line or thoracocentesis, paracentesis, et cetera."

In Singapore, apart from the Duke-NUS Medical School which offers a post-graduate medical degree similar to what David underwent, both the National University of Singapore (NUS) and the Nanyang Technological University (NTU) offer undergraduate medical degrees. Both undergraduate and post-graduate medical training entailed two years of pre-clinical work, followed by three or two years of clinical work, respectively. Medical training in our current era is very protected — both for the patients as well as for medical students. Students generally undergo a period of intense lecture-based curriculum during their pre-clinical years, before embarking on a clinical phase where they dip their hands in a myriad of clinical services offered by the health system. During this latter phase of their training, students are expected to shadow doctors on the wards in hospital, and typically function more as curious observers rather than as functional members of the team. Their hands-on experiences are typically on mannequins and on each other, and only in the twilight of their medical school career do they experience life as a 'sub-intern', colloquially known as the Student Internship Programme (SIP). Even then, the actual procedures performed by them are mostly innocuous, including phlebotomy and inserting cannulas, and all routinely under strict supervision. They would most certainly not be expected to perform lumbar punctures or deliver babies. As much as many of us 'old school' doctors bemoan the lack of experience of the incoming medical fraternity, this approach of gradual embedding of students into the workforce is ultimately important as we strive to balance their needs with that of the safety of the patients.

Naturally for David, his medical education in university prepared him well for the transition to working life. "Those experiences made the transition slightly less stressful. When I began my formal residency as an intern and a medical officer, I was on my way to becoming more efficient with procedures. I had about a one-month head start in the sense of having clinical skills, and similarly for procedural skills. So that was kind of nice."

He shares with us some historical perspectives on medical education, the inevitable path of reinvention it took over the past few decades, and the route which is currently still being refined. "The Sunset Commission ultimately led to the changes that exist now, which are restricted hours that you all have. Those were expropriated from the States as part of ACGME."[5] Like most institutions in Singapore, the traditional training of medical doctors was inherited from our former colonial masters. This basic specialty training/advanced specialty training (BST/AST) system lacked structure, and more crucially, regulation. It was not infrequent that, in the past, doctors training in this system were subjected to working up to 100–120 hours a week. All this came to a halt when Singapore adopted the residency system from the United States back in 2010. At least in principle, training became more organised, and working hours were restricted to a maximum of 80 hours a week.

David continues to explicate. "Some of it is medicolegal issues, some were structural issues with regard to how to balance service versus education during training. A lot of that has been rethought. Essentially, starting in the early- to mid-80s, medical educators began to think of how to improve the educational system. When I was training in Medicine and Infectious Diseases, you learned via high patient volume. It was just relentless. We were on-call every 72 hours and for about 1–2 month each year, every 48 hours. That was part of the rite of passage. Some of it was to deal with the work that needed to be done. However, it also served to break down your wilfulness, your independence, to teach you just to be able to respond at three in the morning, and to do all the things that you needed to do. That led to medical errors, no doubt, from fatigue, and to burnout."

We nod in agreement. We have been through a similar system before, though probably not as inhospitable as it was in David's time. The times when we have to work for thirty hours at a stretch can be mentally and physically challenging, and this was not only detrimental for the doctor, but quite likely for the patients as well. But this debate has been on-going since time immemorial. The corollary of a lack of experience from volume and practice would be that of disservice and possible harm to the patient. Many doctors, especially in Singapore, are now becoming specialists at a precocious age of their training, sometimes as early as five years out of medical school, and it is not uncommon to hear a lament from them about a deficiency of experience.

David gives pause at this moment, reflecting upon all that has happened to medical education which has led us right up to now. Does he agree that the pendulum has now swung to the other extreme? Were we becoming soft in our training of the next generation of doctors and specialists?

"Well, there's no right answer for me to say. I think it has its pros and cons. I think you certainly learn better when you're not chronically fatigued. And you probably have better mental health, because I saw some of my colleagues suffer, and I'm sure I suffered. But I worry about volume. So much of what we do requires exposure in order to learn. And I know, for instance, in some surgical subspecialties, the surgeons that train in the UK or the US have done maybe several hundreds of a particular procedure by the time they finish their training. And in Singapore, they're only able to do a low fraction of that by the time they finish their surgical training due to the finite number of cases and the number of trainees. So I worry about that. But there are pros and cons."

We prod him to share his thoughts on how the current medical education system could improve, but he declines to comment. It probably isn't because he is devoid of ideas. Perhaps the horse has already bolted, and he can only continue to do what he does best, cultivating the next generation at an individual level. We leave the topic at that for now, but at the back of our minds, can we, the next generation of doctors, be trusted to carry the torch?

Notes

[1] Acquired immunodeficiency syndrome. The disease caused by HIV.

[2] Azidothymidine. Also known as zidovudine, the first legally licensed anti-retroviral therapy (ART) used to treat people living with HIV.

[3] Medical Officer. The rank attained by doctors after doing a year of houseman-ship.

[4] Lumbar puncture.

[5] Accreditation Council for Graduate Medical Education

INFECTIOUS DISEASES

–

per aspera ad astra
'through hardships to the stars'

S ince the dawn of the medical profession, infectious syndromes have routinely been encountered by physicians from all walks of life. Managing them was, and still is, a required part of their armamentarium, although the available arsenal prior to the arrival of antibiotics had been limited. Before antibiotics, bloodletting would have been the de facto 'treatment' option for most febrile and inflammatory conditions. The humoral theory was the guiding principle in Western medicine since antiquity right up to the 19th century, with the underlying assumption being that the human body contained four humors (Latin for *'fluids'*) — black bile (melancholy), yellow bile (choler), blood, and phlegm — and imbalances in these resulted in illness. Restoration of health was only achieved once equilibrium was reinstated. Accomplishing this typically involved sweating, diuresis, purging, or bloodletting of the patient, with the latter the most commonly practiced by far. One of its famous victims was the first president of the United States, George Washington, who fatally succumbed to quinsy, but only after having two-fifths of his blood exsanguinated as therapy. In an ironic turn of events, antibiotics are now ubiquitous in the management of fevers, regardless of its underlying pathology. The humoristic theory could only be disproved once the dissection of the human body became less taboo, allowing the intellectual study of the human body, or Anatomy, to take root in medical education, beginning in the 17th century. This in turn permitted the twin pillars of Physiology and Pathology to develop, incorporating a scientific basis towards understanding human health and disease.

Another major concept about disease and contagion bequeathed from classical times was the miasmatic theory. Disease was thought to have arisen from a pathologic atmosphere, such as air contaminated by noxious vapers produced from putrefying matter, and bodies succumbed once exposed to it. The infectious syndrome, malaria, was emblematic of this. The name is derived from '*mal aria*', or '*bad air*' in Italian, where previously it was thought to arise from breathing contaminated air from swamps and rotting vegetation, though now is proven to be caused by the parasite *Plasmodium* transmitted by the bite of an *Anopheles* mosquito. The refutation of the miasma theory arose with the advent of modern Microbiology, in the form of the germ theory, led by Drs Louis Pasteur and Robert Koch. Pasteur disproved, experimentally, the long-held belief that microorganisms spontaneously generated from non-living substances, and Koch demonstrated a link between a disease and a particular microbe, with anthrax and its agent, *Bacillus anthracis*, setting the precedence.

Yet, even before Sir Alexander Fleming's serendipitous discovery of penicillin, the world's first naturally-derived antibiotic, in 1928, fatalities from communicable diseases in industrialized countries were already on the wane since the turn of the 20th century. The Industrial Revolution, which had begun in the late 1700s, had coalesced the rural masses with rapid urbanization, and the subsequent explosion in population density created the ideal conditions for the spread of contagion such as tuberculosis and waterborne diseases. This was eventually curbed by state interventions with the institution of public health measures such as improvements in nutrition, sanitation, living conditions, and medical care. These significantly reduced the burden of infectious diseases in the population — in the States, mortality rates from communicable diseases declined from 600 deaths per 100,000 individuals per year in 1900 to 120 in 1940, and in England and Wales, a similar decline from 550 deaths per 100,000 individuals per year to 130 during the same period was seen.[1] 1941 was the year when penicillin was first prescribed for use on a human patient, and from thenceforth, there was no looking back. What followed after was the golden age of antimicrobial discovery, and together with widespread immunisation and continued improvements in public health practices, infectious syndromes were becoming less frequently encountered by the common practitioner. Just as the management of such conditions became rarefied, individual cases were becoming more complex with the advent of both solid organ and bone marrow transplantation, immunosuppressive therapy, and their concomitant smorgasbord of infections.

Once the use of antibiotics became widespread, it was not long before pathogens developed defences with antimicrobial resistance. The scourge of these multi-drug resistant organisms may come to be one of the biggest problems in the modern era. Treatment of these organisms often requires the use of novel agents or unique combinations of existing antibiotics. With these factors contributing, there came to be recognition of the need for a coterie of physicians with an interest in infectious diseases. This saw the establishment of Infectious Diseases, the specialty, in the late 1960s in the States.[2] In Europe, the specialty was only formally recognised by the European Union of Medical Specialists in 1997, a significant delay due in part to the direct role Clinical Microbiologists continued to play in the management of infectious syndromes.[3] Microbiologists in the US, being scientists by training, were not medically qualified and therefore excluded from dispensing clinical advice.

In the United States, the first batch of ABIM[4] ID Board-certified ID specialists qualified in 1972, and David joined the nascent field as a trainee in 1986, becoming a specialist two years later. How had he decided on ID for a career? It was not an obvious choice of specialty at the time. In fact, soon after the establishment of the entity, the demise of the specialty was prophesied. Dr Robert Petersdorf, ironically an ID physician himself, published an opinion piece in the medical journal, the NEJM,[5] back in 1978, less than a decade after ID had been established.[6] On the backdrop of advances in antimicrobial therapy, widespread immunisation programmes, and improvements in public health, he derisively proclaimed the imminent end of both infectious diseases and its specialist physicians. *'Even with my great personal loyalties to Infectious Disease, I cannot conceive a need for 309 more Infectious-Disease experts unless they spend their time culturing each other.'* And yet, David chose to join this apparently imminently sinking ship. Was it naivety, or prescience?

"I know this quote very well. ID came from Immunologists, they came from Paediatricians, they came from Microbiologists. Physicians migrated from a variety of different fields and eventually became the Infectious Diseases practitioners of the future. I knew the milieu from where he [Robert Petersdorf] came from." This was Boston. "I'd never met Petersdorf myself, but I was involved in arranging for speakers from his department and others to speak during our medical grand rounds, and for some of our other educational programmes when I was responsible for arranging those. My training was after he had made his statement regarding the future of ID — I was still in undergraduate school at that time the article was published."

He pares the issue down to the bone. Fundamentally, it was just hubris and karma. "These kinds of absolutes always go back and bite you on the bottom, right? People who basically say this with such arrogance and authority..." He subtly reproaches his predecessors for being blindsided. "There was a lack of looking beyond the boundaries that existed at the time. I wasn't worried about not having a job. I began post-graduate medical training at the beginning of the AIDS pandemic, and there was clearly a need for many more ID physicians. And at the time, there were only a couple of thousands in the country. The universe of need grows, and will continue to grow. I was not fearful of not having a job."

He elaborates. "Since I've become an Infectious Diseases specialist, the niches of antibiotic stewardship, infection prevention and control, and transplant ID have expanded dramatically. All these areas including HIV care have expanded their need for ID physicians. When we tried to prepare for this pandemic [COVID-19[7]], we were not prepared despite our efforts. How can we prepare for the next pandemic?" He had a tone of indignance. The answer was rhetorical. "We need to expand our capacity in anticipation of future need. Examples of instances where there are too many ID physicians for the work required are rare."

You can hear a certain weariness in his voice, borne over the decades from trying to convince various stakeholders on the value that our specialty brings. In his universe, there can't be enough of a good thing, the good thing being ID specialists. Having ID specialists abound is beneficial to the medical ecosystem — consultations by them have been shown to save costs and reduce patient in-hospital mortality.[8] Frustratingly, we are a dying breed,[9] and we are partially the cause of our own demise. Chiefly, we straddle across two worlds — the microscopic and the macroscopic — and as it is, learning about humans is complex enough, let alone with the addition of pathogens. We kick ourselves in the teeth with overcomplicated names for both our therapies and our 'adversaries' — tongue-twisters such as ibrexafungerp or fosmanogepix, two of the latest antifungal therapies, or *Orientia tsutsugamushi*, a mite-borne bacterium that causes scrub typhus in humans, do us no favours at all. Our range of knowledge has to be sweeping — familiarity with geography is indispensable, keeping abreast with current affairs is a prerequisite, and acquaintanceship with all bodily organ systems is vital. As a maxim, infectious diseases know no boundaries. There's no money to be made — we are one of the lowest paid specialties worldwide,[9] and the community we serve generally do not encompass rich folks. Our specialty may kill us, or have certain stigmas associated with it — from handling patients with the deadliest organisms such as Ebolavirus to multi-drug resistant tuberculosis, to caring for the outcasts from the lepers to those with sexually transmitted infections. These are what we may encounter throughout our career, and it requires a certain humility to do the job. But there is no doubt that we can be haughty too. We hold the purse-strings for one of the most commonly used drugs on the planet — antibiotics — and we can be pretty acerbic when they are being misused. Only because we know what's best for the patient (we jest). But he's preaching to the converted.

To understand why David had chosen to be an ID physician, although potentially both oversimplified and melodramatic, one could pinpoint the 6th and 8th of August 1945 as pivotal moments. Hiroshima and Nagasaki and the first times nuclear weapons were unleashed on humanity. The first group of victims perished immediately from the physical effects of the blast, but a second group soon followed in the coming days and weeks, a result of the atom's effects on the cell. Unbeknownst to physicians and scientists back then, these victims had succumbed to acute radiation sickness, which wiped out the body's haematopoietic stem cells, the multipotent precursor cells with the ability to regenerate all cell types of the blood. With their bone marrow annihilated, these victims were left vulnerable to infections and haemorrhage to which they eventually succumbed. Medical research stemming from the atomic bomb eventually led to the dawn of bone marrow transplantation, a life-changing procedure that has since been used to cure a myriad of conditions, including blood disorders and cancers such as leukaemia, and in exceptionally unique cases, persons living with HIV. In a bizarre way, this makes J. Robert Oppenheimer, also known as the Father of the atomic bomb, the Grandfather of bone marrow transplantation.

To be clear, David's heart had not always been on Infectious Diseases. Instead, he had wanted to follow in the footsteps of a fellow Texan and the founding Father of bone marrow transplantation, Professor E. Donnall 'Don' Thomas. "I thought, following on the intellectual rigor when I trained in Internal Medicine, I went to New York with the explicit anticipation of becoming a Bone Marrow Transplanter. That's what I wanted to do. As I went into Medicine, the specialties Gastroenterology and Cardiology had just been born. I knew I wanted to be a subspecialist. I wasn't interested in outpatient medicine. I wanted to be where the action was."

It feels almost blasphemous to us, that the Father of ID in Singapore almost was not. His interest in bone marrow transplantation was simple — because it was complex. "Because I thought that was the coolest thing in the world. We were gaining understanding of fundamental immunology issues at the time as a result of HIV. And I was so fascinated by the opportunistic infections that arose. I thought, '*Okay, what would result in the equivalent of HIV or worse on someone's host defence? Wipe out their bone marrow. We get rid of neutrophils, we interfere with immunoglobulin, and if we give ATG,*[10] *we knock out T cells (a type of white blood cell).*' I thought if I could manage the complications associated with that scenario, then that would not only help those transplanted but also be a test of clinical skill."

Once again, this all goes back to the atomic bomb. Blood cancers such as leukaemia do not reside in a particular area of the body, unlike solid organ malignancies. The latter can be excised from the body, or have radiotherapy targeted to its specific location, as treatment. Not so the former, being fluid in nature. Ionizing radiation from the atomic bomb was shown to obliterate the bone marrow, and could, in principle, be utilised as treatment for blood cancers, only that the cure was worse than the disease. You would not survive long without your blood cells. And that's where the restorative power of bone marrow transplantation comes in, and that's why Professor Don Thomas' work won him the Nobel Prize in Medicine in 1990. And about David, you could say he loved picking up the pieces more than pressing the detonator.

"I wanted to do transplant. But then the transplanters at Sloan Kettering and New York Hospital at that time were generally quite arrogant. They were really full of themselves, and rightfully so. They were very smart people, published a tonne, and were moving the field forward. But you couldn't sit in a room without wanting to hit them." His sentiments have similarly been echoed by some of our hospital's senior Haematologists who have encountered that generation of overseas transplanters during their attachments abroad. That kind of behaviour now, hopefully, belonged in the past.

By contrast, he found that he admired the ones who did ID. "The ID physicians were confident yet cool. Their pants were too short, and they all wore pocket protectors. But I thought, '*Okay. That's all right. That's just part of the gang signs.*' They were all very bright, and the logic was there. So this was what appealed to me, Infectious Diseases." It was *déjà vu*, a replay of his earlier educational switch from Oceanography to Medicine. There were a few important lessons for us to glean from these two episodes. Firstly, be rid of the 'sunk cost fallacy' — you need to be honest with yourself, and not be fixated on the initial path chosen, believing that you had to stick to your original commitment. The Chinese idiom, '削足适履', [xuē zú shì lǚ], elucidates it better — '*to shave one's feet to fit one's shoes*'. Secondly, time is not wasted if you have a mid-training/career switch. In fact, both the tangible and intangible skill sets gained may potentially put you in good stead for your next phase in life.

And so began David's training in ID. "I trained at New York Hospital and Hospital for Special Surgery in Manhattan, New York, which was also my Internal Medicine training ground. They were the primary teaching hospitals for Cornell University's medical school. I spent some of my elective time as a 3rd year Medicine resident on the ID service. The transition to being an ID Fellow was smooth. The ID Fellows [the equivalent of a senior resident (SR) or registrar in Singapore] also rotated to Memorial Sloan Kettering Hospital, across the street from New York Hospital. Memorial Sloan Kettering had their own ID programme, but we spent about a quarter of each year in each other's hospitals. Henry W. Murray was the ID Head of Department (HOD) during my time. R. Gordon Douglas, Jr. was Head of Medicine, and he was an ID physician as well. R. Gordon Douglas, Jr. had been ID HOD before ascending to Head of Medicine. He subsequently became President of IDSA,[11] and was an initial editor of '*Mandell, Douglas, and Bennett's Principles and Practice of Infectious Diseases*'." This was *the* indispensable ID textbook of every practicing trainee and specialist.

We exchanged notes on our training curriculum. "The workload was moderate-to-high but manageable. I don't recall having as many conferences in which to present, as occurs in Singapore — but it may be that there are so many more SRs I engage with here that it seems there are more. I would go to my Rockefeller University laboratory, 400 metres from the hospital, starting at 8 AM until 2 PM, then return to the hospital to round on my inpatients and do 'blue letters',[12] then round with other ID attendings, then round on the late-rounding ID physician's private patients before he finished his clinic. Then we'd swing by the Microbiology laboratory and Radiology department to make eye contact with our colleagues and share relevant case nuances with the Microbiologists and Radiologists. Then I would meet the late-rounding attending to round with him on his patients for one-on-one teaching from 7 or 8 PM until we finished, sometimes around midnight, then have a late dinner one to two nights a week with him near the hospital. I would stay in hospital until 12 to 1 AM on most weekdays." That sounds neither like a moderate-to-high nor manageable work load. "On weekends, I was either on ID service, or in the Rockefeller laboratory. Or moonlighting. I was paid US$ 16,000/year as an ID Fellow." It seemed like he had neither time nor money.

Next, we compared the tools of our trade. "We did the Gram stains and smears on the ward. We had chocolate agar plates and small incubators on the wards so that we could immediately plate and incubate urethral swabs, so that they didn't run into problems on the way to the lab. As a trainee, we didn't have polymerase chain reaction (PCR) tests. We had serologies, and we had some antigen detection tests available, so that wasn't terribly different compared with today." We weren't so sure about that. Firstly, none of the ID trainees in our local context were fluent in performing rudimentary microbiological tests nor manipulating a microscope. We could definitely wield a stethoscope. Secondly, PCRs were crucial components of our diagnostic toolkit. In our current day and age, PCRs are utilised for a wide range of infectious syndromes, from respiratory tract infections to meningitis to joint infections to gastroenteritis. The world we practiced in *was* very different today.

He continues to describe what seemed like the prehistoric times of Medicine to us. "Things that we didn't have diagnostics for, we made clinical diagnoses. But I would do a Tzanck prep to diagnose HSV.[13] I was expected to do LPs and do my Gram stain, and then I'd have the answer. Because you couldn't wait for the Microbiologist. We had a dedicated sink where everything splashed. We even mixed chemotherapy on the ward. Pharmacy would deliver anthracyclines and I'm there mixing it, and you'll get blisters on your hand." It sounded like trench warfare to us, though this was just the everyday life of a trainee back in those days.

"But back then, what else was I going to do? Wait for the *Listeria*[14] to grow? No. I mean, you needed something to go by. You had to have some discernment. It was considered inelegant to treat everybody for everything. Because you had to defend your management decisions, no matter who you were. You were the resident. You have to say why we did this. The big revolution was when HSV PCR became available for CSF,[15] because before that, we were doing stereotactic biopsies of people's temporal lobes, and that was never satisfying." Just to qualify, he had never been required to perform those. They had been rightfully left in the hands of the neurosurgeons.

To make matters worse, a lack of appropriate diagnostics was compounded by a lack of effective therapy. "It was unnerving. Because when I first arrived in New York from Texas, when I was a houseman, acyclovir had not been invented yet." This is our current standard anti-viral therapy for HSV infections. "It came when I was a third-year resident. We had ara-A[16] and ara-C[17] which were antiviral agents. But ara-A had less bone marrow toxicity, and was more effective against HSV. Although it required huge volumes of free water to go into solution, so everybody we infused it in developed hyponatraemia. You did not want to have HSV encephalitis back then."

We do a rapid-fire question-and-answer segment next to ascertain the differences in practice across the generations. One good gauge was to establish the antimicrobial resistance profiles of commonly encountered pathogens, and how broad the spectrum of coverage the antibiotics utilised were. One of the reasons why the opinions of ID physicians are so highly sought after is because, over the years, the treatment of pathogens has become significantly more complicated as pathogens become more resistant to antimicrobial therapies. This entailed utilizing ever expensive and expansive drugs with increasingly convoluted names.

The most commonly used antimicrobials in medical practice belong to the β-lactam group of antibiotics, and penicillin would be included in this category. They all contain the core β-lactam structure within their molecule. One of the ways bacteria circumvent this is to produce enzymes which hydrolyse this β-lactam ring and render it ineffective, and the first resistant bacteria were found to produce such enzymes, termed β-lactamases. In a tit-for-tat move, scientists further came up with antibiotics which were impervious to break down by these enzymes, and hence were more broad-spectrum in their coverage, only to encounter the rise of more resistance in the form of extended-spectrum β-lactamases (ESBLs). As the Red Queen told Alice in Lewis Carroll's *'Through the Looking-Glass'*, *'it takes all the running you can do, to keep in the same place'*, this microscopic warfare is essentially the Red Queen hypothesis played out in real life — bacteria and humans must continually evolve new adaptations (antimicrobial resistance in bacteria, and antibiotics by humans) so as to avoid extinction. The problem with this escalating conflict is that these pathogens reproduce and mutate faster than humans can come up with new ammunitions, and we are now living on the cusp of a post-antibiotic era. Bacteria containing ESBLs are now routinely encountered in our everyday practice — we wouldn't bat an eyelid seeing one. We start off with a low bar — were bacteria with ESBLs a common occurrence back when he started out?

"No."

That line of pursuit ended much faster than expected. There was not much antimicrobial resistance encountered during his apprenticeship. In the hierarchy of β-lactam antimicrobial resistance, there were β-lactamases, then ESBLs, then *AmpC* β-lactamases, and then there were carbapenemases. The latter are notoriously difficult to treat with limited antimicrobial options available. What were the heavy-weight antibiotics that he otherwise employed back then?

"My top gun was ticarcillin. I also had piperacillin-tazobactam, ceftazidime, and quinolones." These would have been antibiotics used to treat *Pseudomonas*, a particularly pesky healthcare-associated pathogen. "This was when I was a Fellow. I had access to echinocandins at the end of my fellowship. I had fluconazole. But I gave intravenous ketoconazole earlier on before fluconazole was available. Amphotericin B was a mainstay in the empiric management of neutropenic fever and established invasive moulds. I had chloramphenicol." Alas, some of these were either obsolete, or were run-of-the-mill antimicrobials that we, presently, all too frequently utilised, some of them as our first-line drug of choice. Apart from echinocandins which are relatively broad-spectrum anti-fungal therapies, the rest were like pistols in this era, and far from being our top gun. Moving on to infectious syndromes — how were pneumonias treated?

"Cefoxitin or cefotetan was given. When we identified pneumococcus, we gave penicillin, but only if it was community-acquired. We would almost always give a macrolide of some sort. At the time, it was intravenous erythromycin, and that burned everybody's veins."

How about urinary tract infections?

"Nitrofurantoin for cystitis. Cephalothin or cefazolin for pyelonephritis. We also had cotrimoxazole."

In this era, the bacteria that we oftentimes encountered were all too frequently resistant to the narrow-spectrum antibiotics deployed during the nascent years of our specialty. This issue of antimicrobial resistance will be revisited again later in the interview, and it may all be rhetorical, but we do not know how much road we have left to run.

We return back to issues about training. The beginnings of one's training in ID can be particularly daunting, with a steep learning curve and a bevy of patients, and trainees typically feel overwhelmed when starting out. Had he faced similar growing pains?

"There were two or three senior consultants who were enthusiastic mentors and eager to engage if one showed interest. We were given latitude to run our ID service, either 'blue letters' or as the primary team, with independence and the trust that we'd seek input as indicated. Some attending ID physicians were more hands on, some hands off. It was motivation to get 'up to speed' quickly. I never felt abandoned as I had the confidence I could find the answer in the literature and if not, seek their input."

What was his approach, then, to learning as a fledgling ID trainee?

"Seeking and learning fundamental concepts of microbe pathogenicity, host defence, host vulnerability, modifiers of host and pathogen phenotypes, and then all these aspects combined to anticipate host-pathogen interaction. With these concepts, it can be relatively straightforward adding new findings or observations to the paradigms to either re-enforce existing understanding or modify it accordingly." These all came naturally to him, this mastery of the subject, though not so for others. He had, and still has, his gripes though. "The manner in which fundamental information is organised could be annoying, however. For example, I found, and still find, some of the disorganised and sometimes overlapping systems for microbial nomenclature challenging when trying to teach with clarity."

Just as David has been an inspiring mentor to us, we were curious if there was anyone who played a similar role for him.

"A man by the name of Donald Armstrong. He's an Infectious Diseases physician, an old school guy. I think he's definitely retired." We look it up and he, unfortunately, passed on in November 2018. The late Dr Donald Armstrong was the first Director of the Microbiology laboratory at Memorial Sloan Kettering, and subsequently the first Chief of the Infectious Diseases services in 1971. "He was a past President of the Infectious Disease Society of

America. He was a Head of Infectious Diseases at Memorial Sloan Kettering. He had long hair, a full head of hair. I knew him when he was already old. He did mostly transplant work. He'd done a lot of the early work with neutropenic fever, and was engaged with his Fellows in doing good clinical research, and encouraged quite a few to do basic research. And he was passionate about social issues. And I saw him as a bit of a Renaissance man. He was smart as a whip, very bright, and very passionate. He read a lot. And so, he was my kind of a good ID guy." And then, he seemingly recalls an old joke and takes a swing at his idol and the specialty as a whole. "But you know, to be a good ID guy…let's be honest…doesn't take a huge amount."

He jests, surely. His recorded words state otherwise. David himself once commented that ID physicians were invaluable, and all had certain characteristics — we had a good fund of knowledge of General Medicine, and a very good working knowledge of the subspecialties of Internal Medicine; we had good problem-solving skills, were curious, perseverant, had a high threshold for tolerance, were attentive and observant; we had to be skilled communicators, diplomats and debaters; and we had to be organised and have an interest in teaching.[18] He promises to let us in on the joke later. But first, we get him to flesh out the details. Surely there had to be more to Dr Donald Armstrong?

"I thought he functioned well, and he was humble. At the old ICAAC,[19] which is called ID Week now, he gave one of the plenary talks. He didn't talk about ID at all. He talked about the amount of money being spent on the military industrial complex in the United States. That was a talk. I was like, '*This is cool*'. Because he saw it as his role as an Infectious Diseases physician, as a leader in the Infectious Diseases community, to tell us we have responsibilities beyond taking care of the next pneumonia, that we should aspire to more than that. Not that it's not good enough, but we should want to optimize our utility to society."

David, however, qualifies. "He wasn't my direct boss. I interacted with him. I was at Cornell and Rockefeller and I would go do time at Memorial Sloan Kettering. Also, some of my basic research was at Sloan Kettering. So, I interfaced with him, and plus we're literally across the street, and there was a lot of inbreeding between the two programmes. He had his own group of

Fellows, but each year I spent time with him. And then, even when I wasn't there, I was 'around' them." Being in the same zip code, he was essentially cooking in the same broth despite not being under the same umbrella.

He summarizes. "It was just the way he carried himself, the way he saw his duty. He was not stern. He didn't take himself so seriously. He was a very approachable, nice man who was capable." One could very well say the same about David.

We bring up another topic that was dear to many ID physicians — HIV. If the dawn of transplantation and immunosuppression saw the star of Infectious Diseases rising, it was HIV which cemented its day in the sun. The history of HIV is well known to the ID community — in 1981, the journal Morbidity and Mortality Weekly Report (MMWR) published a case series about a group of patients with *Pneumocystis carinii* (now known as *Pneumocystis jirovecii*) pneumonia in Los Angeles, California.[20] This fungus typically caused pneumonia in patients with a defunct immunity, and it turned out to be the first publication on what was subsequently known as acquired immunodeficiency syndrome (AIDS). Since the start of the epidemic, up to 85 million people have been infected by the virus, and around 40 million have died from AIDS-related illnesses.[21] Before COVID-19 came along, HIV was *the* archetypal ID disease. It came from our closest relatives, the chimpanzees, in the emerald forests of central Africa; because of its capacity for latency, it insidiously ravaged through its human host, and humanity as a whole, before unsuspectingly rearing its ugly head to become both disfiguring and devastating; it afflicted, and still continues to afflict, the ostracized and the marginalised; and it was fatal, at least before the advent of anti-retroviral therapy (ART), and still remains incurable. What was it like for David as a professional practicing so near the epicentre where the epidemic was first uncovered?

"I was a 3rd year medical student in Dallas, Texas, in June 1981, when the initial MMWR articles were published. The implications were not clear to me then. The syndrome was described on the US coasts, New York and San Francisco, but was identified in Dallas a month or two later. At that time, it was described in MSM[22] and women involved in IDU,[23] sex work and their children only, later in Haitians and haemophiliacs. The syndrome wasn't called AIDS, but 'severe immune deficiency'. In early 1982, the syndrome was briefly given the name GRID,[24] and in late 1982, 'AIDS' was coined. I was fascinated, but at that time, all human pathophysiology and how different individuals and different societies and subcultures dealt with illness and mortality fascinated me." This was the anthropological side of him speaking.

At the beginning of the epidemic, no one knew what the cause of the disease was, how it spread, how it could be detected, and how it could be treated. Crucially, no one knew how to define it — it presented in a multitude of ways, from a fever to diarrhoea to severe pneumonia to leukaemia to early-onset dementia, and a patient could have all of these at once. Anyone seeking healthcare could potentially be harbouring it. It preyed upon the deepest fears of the medical fraternity, that they could catch an undetectable, untreatable, unsurvivable deadly contagion from their patients — so much so that patients with certain 'traits', such as those mentioned by David earlier, were actively denied medical care by a portion of medical practitioners.[25] Before its mode of transmission was determined — either through sexual contact, blood products, needles, or from mother-to-infant — everyone adopted extreme measures when seeing such patients, wearing total body gowns with gloves, goggles and masks.[26] What had it truly been like, down on the ground?

"I noticed nothing odd in Dallas — this may have been my limited perspective at that time. By 1983 we knew it spread by needles, amongst MSM, and via blood products. It was not clear at that time why women were less impacted. By 1984, as women not involved with IDU or sex trade were increasingly identified as PWAs,[27] it then became clear. As a medical intern in 1983, I was expected to pursue patient questioning regarding CMV,[28] amyl nitrates, and a variety of off-target issues, trying to identify an aetiology or aetiologies for AIDS before the retrovirus was discovered." The virus was eventually identified in May 1983 by Luc Montagnier from the Pasteur Institute in Paris, and even that had its controversies.[29] Beyond its effect on the healthcare system, society on the whole was equally transformed. "The free-wheeling social atmosphere in Manhattan had been somewhat muted since the 1981 reports, and it was further impacted when heterosexual transmission was recognised."

"When I moved to New York for Internal Medicine residency, followed by ID training, I had to deal with uninformed professional behaviour. Nurses were professional and, in general, did not hesitate to provide care. Surgeons and other interventionalists in many hospitals were less consistent. The more informed took appropriate precautions and went about their business. However, some refused to care for PWAs. This was readily addressed — if you refused to care for HIV-infected individuals in a professional manner, then you were not referred any cases at all. This impacted your ability to teach, generate revenue, et cetera. We briefly directed all cases, HIV and otherwise, to the informed proceduralists or threatened to send all the non-PWA cases needing procedures to a nearby hospital. While this didn't change hearts, it changed minds. Winning hearts took longer. ID physicians were happy to be in the centre of attention of the academic universe — grants eventually flowed, trials flourished, more money meant more faculty and support staff. It was a deep vein to mine."

Did he similarly experience fear during that period?

"I was never scared. Maybe it was youth, but I was never worried about HIV. I thought, naively or not, that understanding the things we were exposed to would allow me to protect myself and my loved ones. Was I ever fearful for my life? I stabbed myself with an 18-gauge needle after taking bloods from somebody who had uncontrolled HIV when I was a house officer. That was before the era of antiretrovirals. So that was a little anxiety provoking. Things went well." He adds in a little quip. "That said, I did acquire tuberculosis from the hospital." These were the professional hazards we faced when managing infectious diseases on a routine basis, and '*a little anxiety*' was definitely downplaying the dread and the fear that many of us experience whilst we await the all clear from our blood test. This could be up to a nerve-wrecking six months from the exposure.

Many of us working in the healthcare setting find it rewarding because of the ability to make a difference in a person's life so tangibly. Functional cure with highly active antiretroviral therapy (HAART) only came about in 1996, more than a decade after the epidemic first broke out in the States. Prior to that, a diagnosis of AIDS was a definite death sentence. What was the feeling like knowing that there was nothing one could do for their patient?

"On the one hand, helpless. On the other hand, if you stepped back and thought about it — it allowed you to be what doctors have always been historically, privileged to witness and journey with fellow humans when they are most vulnerable. To provide physical and emotional solace, as able. To support our patients when others had abandoned them. To provide our patients the recognition, dignity and humanity we all deserve." An aphorism commonly ascribed to both Dr Edward Livingston Trudeau and Hippocrates unveils this truth about the duties of a doctor — '*to cure sometimes, to relieve often, to comfort always.*' Stripped down to its core, doctors are meant to be a patient's advocate. He concludes. "The HIV pandemic was a net positive for the specialty due to the professionalism and selflessness displayed by the majority of our ID colleagues."

We wrap up this segment by discussing his transition from trainee to consultant. This is usually a source of mixed feelings for many doctors — on one hand, we were elated to have cleared the bar to become independent practitioners in our chosen field, but on the other, it was a time of fraught as this was when the buck stopped at us. We were expected to know what was best for our patients; and they and the medical team we led all looked to us for answers. How was it like for David?

"I felt excellent. I felt Infectious Diseases better utilised my skillset compared to a focus limited to General Internal Medicine. I embraced this burden of responsibility. I enjoyed, and still enjoy, the daily challenges, the strategies to value uncertainty as a variable in decision making, and refining the tools needed to communicate occasionally abstract concepts. I ran towards this burden." Once again, this was typical David — indomitable and devil-may-care. These were hard footsteps to follow in.

We return back to the joke he had promised to let us in on — why wasn't it *that* hard to become an ID physician?

"My Head of Department, then R. Gordon Douglas, told me that, '*You can teach a monkey to do ID in three months.*' I said, '*Then why is my training three years?*'"

David chuckles ahead of the punchline.

"'*You're not as smart as a monkey.*'"

We definitely did not see that one coming.

Notes

[1] OECD. 'Stemming the Superbug Tide. Just a Few Dollars More', *OECD Health Policy Studies*, OECD Publishing, Paris 2018.

[2] E. H. Kass. 'History of the specialty of infectious diseases in the United States', *Ann Intern Med*, 1987 May;106(5):745–56.

[3] F. J. Cooke et al. 'Postgraduate training in infectious diseases: investigating the current status in the international community', *Lancet Infect Dis*. 2005 Jul;5(7):440–9.

[4] American Board of Internal Medicine

[5] New England Journal of Medicine

[6] R. G. Petersdorf. 'The doctors' dilemma', *N Engl J Med*. 1978 Sep 21;299(12):628–34.

[7] Coronavirus disease 2019

[8] M. Sasikumar et al. 'The value of specialist care-infectious disease specialist referrals-why and for whom? A retrospective cohort study in a French tertiary hospital', *Eur J Clin Microbiol Infect Dis*, 2017 Apr;36(4):625–633.

[9] T. H. Swartz et al. 'Preserving the Future of Infectious Diseases: Why We Must Address the Decline in Compensation for Clinicians and Researchers', *Clin Infect Dis*, 2023 Nov 17;77(10):1387–1394.

[10] Anti-thymocyte globulin

[11] Infectious Diseases Society of America

[12] A colloquial term in the Singapore medical system for referrals. Before electronic health records took hold of our lives, referrals made by the treating team to specialists were written on blue-coloured paper, hence the term 'blue letter'.

[13] Herpes simplex virus

[14] *Listeria* is an organism that typically causes meningoencephalitis in the extremes of ages, as well as those with a defective immunity. Empiric antibiotic coverage for this infectious syndrome, meningoencephalitis, typically did not cover for *Listeria* unless you fell into those risk groups.

[15] Cerebrospinal fluid

[16] Vidarabine or adenine arabinoside

[17] Cytarabine or cytosine arabinoside

[18] Dr David Allen (SG50 Interview) [https://youtu.be/eShvR0OHiE8?si=tBdwF4QbEP1d-Bl] (accessed 31 Jan 2024)

[19] Interscience Conference on Antimicrobial Agents and Chemotherapy

[20] CDC. '*Pneumocystis* pneumonia—Los Angeles', *MMWR Morb Mortal Wkly Rep.* 1981 Jun 5;30(21):250–2.

[21] UNAIDS. 'World AIDS Day 2023: Fact Sheet' [https://www.unaids.org/sites/default/files/media_asset/UNAIDS_FactSheet_en.pdf] (accessed 31 Jan 2024)

[22] Men who have sex with men

[23] Injecting drug users

[24] Gay-related immune deficiency. This was, unfortunately, a deplorable name given for the condition because of its association with homosexual men. It did nothing but stigmatize the very people who needed help.

[25] B. Gerbert et al. 'Why Fear Persists: Health Care Professionals and AIDS', *JAMA.* 1988;260(23):3481–3483

[26] T. N. DeVita. 'Fighting a Plague: Doctors' Stories of Challenge and Innovation Combatting the AIDS Epidemic in 1980s New York City', *J Hist Med Allied Sci.* 2022 Jun 14;77(3):316–342.

[27] People with AIDS

[28] Cytomegalovirus

[29] Robert Gallo, a retrovirus expert from the National Cancer Institute in Bethesda, similarly claimed to have identified the virus causing AIDS in 1983, and had developed a test for its detection. However, pictures of the virus he had broadcasted at a news conference were identical to images of Luc Montagnier's virus. The two had, prior to this, teamed up to research on this new infectious entity, but Gallo had failed to credit his collaborator. Eventually, after years of dispute and negotiations, Montagnier and Gallo agreed, in 1987, to share the spoils.

SINGAPORE

—

e pluribus unum

'out of many, one'

Singapore has been no slouch in the global fight against infectious diseases.

In February 1957, in an all too familiar story about pandemic origins, a novel virus causing respiratory illness emerged from the Guizhou Province of southwestern China. At that stage, the world was still reeling from two World Wars, aggravated during the interbellum years by the deadliest influenza pandemic (the 'Spanish flu' of 1918–1919) in history, and the Great Depression. After ravaging the residents of Hong Kong in the following months, this yet unidentified virus continued its intercontinental march unhindered and unabated, hitching a ride on the global transportation system. It subsequently made landfall in Singapore in May 1957, and it was here that the virus was first isolated, with identification made in collaboration with laboratories abroad. Locally, the investigative and scientific work was led by the Microbiologist, Prof Lim Kok Ann, who was also Singapore's first national chess champion, and his team at the University of Malaya. It was a new strain of influenza A virus of the H2N2[1] subtype. More specifically, it was the influenza A/Singapore/1/1957 (H2N2) — the first strain, belonging to a new subtype of influenza A, identified here, in Singapore.[2] Colloquially, it became known as the 'Singapore flu' or the 'Asian flu'. The pandemic concluded the following year, but not before taking at least a million lives along with it.[3] The H2N2 influenza A virus itself eventually faded out of existence a decade later, only to be replaced by another pandemic-causing influenza A virus of the H3N2 subtype (the 'Hong Kong flu' of 1968–1970).

Before the polio vaccine's incorporation into our national immunisation programme in 1962, outbreaks caused by the poliovirus were a frequent occurrence here in Singapore. At one devastating end of its disease spectrum, the virus caused permanent flaccid paralysis of the limbs in the afflicted. As a matter of trivia, the iron lung, one of the earliest contraptions of artificial ventilation and a precursor to the mechanical ventilators used in our modern-day intensive care units, was specifically developed to manage patients who had respiratory compromise when their breathing muscles were affected by the infection.[4] Two forms of polio vaccines exist — the inactivated poliovirus vaccine (IPV), which was developed by Dr Jonas Salk and licensed in 1955, and the attenuated live-virus oral poliovirus vaccine (OPV), which was developed by Dr Albert Sabin and licensed in 1961. In 1958, just a year after the 'Asian flu' pandemic, Singapore was struck by a polio epidemic, caused by the poliovirus type 1. At that point in time, the OPV existed as a monovalent vaccine made from the type 2 virus, and its use had yet to gain traction due in large part by the success of the IPV in the United States. In collaboration with Dr Albert Sabin, there was sufficient evidence to dictate that the type 2 virus vaccine could provide immunity against the type 1 virus, and a decision was taken by the local medical authorities, led by Dr Ernest Steven Monteiro, to utilise the OPV to stem the outbreak.[5] This was a controversial decision as the OPV had yet to be tested out in the field, though ultimately, this vaccination campaign proved to be a success on two fronts. First of all, it significantly reduced the risk of paralytic disease during the outbreak; secondly, it contributed to the growing body of evidence of the safety and efficacy of the OPV prior to its licensing approval. Singapore has, since October 2000, been certified polio-free by the World Health Organization, and vaccinations have played an outsized role in this.

Prior to 1946, the most commonly prescribed therapy for the treatment of pulmonary tuberculosis, if you could afford it, would have been fresh air brought about by a change of scenery, and better nutrition.[6] Back then, the chances of surviving consumption (which tuberculosis was more widely known as), were not more predictable than the flip of a coin. The first ever randomised control trial, the research tool that has since become a stalwart in the scientific arena, was utilised to determine the efficacy of the antibiotic, streptomycin, in the treatment of pulmonary tuberculosis.[7] It worked, proving to be the first antibiotic effective against tuberculosis, until it did not, when the bacteria eventually developed resistance towards the drug, when it was used as a single agent for therapy. Over the following four decades, the British Medical Research Council conducted multiple clinical trials globally to ascertain the most effective anti-tuberculous regimen. Singapore and the Singapore Tuberculosis Service contributed significantly to this, whether it was in determining the ineffectiveness of the antibiotic thiacetazone as therapy[8] (for which Prof Paul Tambyah's father, Dr John Tambyah, had been one of the medical officers [MO] on the research team), or the role of intermittent dosing of antibiotics in treatment,[9] or in determining the minimum duration of therapy of 6 months for pulmonary infections with drug-susceptible tuberculosis.[10] This was how anti-tuberculosis treatment evolved to the way it is now dispensed, from a single- to a four-drug treatment regimen, with the shortening of the duration of treatment from 24 to 6 months, and Singapore was in the thick of things.[11]

On the local front, nation building post-independence had the inadvertent consequence of reducing communicable diseases.

Resettling Singaporeans from the riverside slums into public housing, or more affectionately known as Housing Development Board (HDB) flats, beyond providing a roof over their heads, was deemed crucial by the government of the day in ensuring that every Singaporean had a stake in the country.[12] On hindsight, this had been pivotal for the control of tuberculosis. The disease, prior to that, was rife in the congested shophouses packed with labourers, which only eased its spread whilst hindering its monitoring and control. Resettlement helped break the chain of transmission by improving living conditions as well as facilitating contact tracing, and together with medical reforms such as compulsory treatment and childhood vaccination, tuberculosis numbers on the island waned. In fact, the Ministry of Health (MOH) eventually concluded that '*perhaps more than any other non-specific measure, this [the resettlement into HDB flats] has played a key role in the reduction of tuberculosis in Singapore*'.[13]

The relocation of itinerant street hawkers into hawker centres and markets was a result of the 1950 Hawkers Inquiry Commission, which had deemed them '*a public nuisance to be removed from the streets*'.[14] Street hawking obstructed the roads, and the indiscriminate disposal of waste together with unsanitary practices was linked to food-borne outbreaks and the proliferation of pests. Licensing and relocation of hawkers to hawker centres began in earnest in 1968, which improved hygiene practices whilst maintaining culinary experiences. It is now more common to see imported cases of cholera or typhoid rather than local ones, with unsavoury practices now confined to the past.[15]

The befouling of our rivers was the impetus for the government to phase out pig farming, beginning in the mid-1980s. Though still an economically viable trade then, it was resource-intensive, highly pollutive, and thus condemned as unsustainable in our metamorphosis into a first world country.[16] Up till then, more than a million pigs were farmed island-wide, producing all the pork needed for local consumption, and more.[17] Along with its demise, a corollary of this was the elimination of Japanese encephalitis (JE) in the island state. In JE, inflammation of the brain is caused by a relative of the dengue virus, the JE virus. The *Culex* mosquitoes are the vectors of this virus, and pigs are one of its animal reservoirs, which complicates eradication of the disease. JE had been endemic in the country up to that point, causing on average more than 10 cases a year, but it subsequently faded out of existence once pig farms were phased out.[18] Currently, the JE virus is found in wild boars on an offshore island,[19] as well as certain farm animals and birds in the peripheral parts of Singapore.[20] Cases of human infection remain sporadic as a result of this intervention.

The eminent 19th century German physician Dr Rudolf Virchow once commented, '*Medicine is a social science and politics is nothing else but medicine on a large scale.*' Singapore's rags-to-riches tale was proof of this — governmental policies and interventions in the daily lives of Singaporeans, unwittingly or not, brought about tremendous gains in public health. Yet, if infectious diseases were being consigned to the history books, why was

Infectious Diseases the specialty still being sought after? Why had David been brought in?

Thus, we began this next section of the interview with a bait. A quote lifted from Dr Victor Heiser's biography, '*An American Doctor's Odyssey*'[21] — '*disease never stays at home in its natural breeding places of filth, but is ever and again breaking into the precincts of its more cleanly neighbours. As long as the Oriental was allowed to remain disease-ridden, he was a constant threat to the Occidental who clung to the idea that he could keep himself healthy in a small disease-ringed circle.*' A fellow American compatriot of the early 20th century, Dr Heiser was a former Associate Director of the International Health division of the Rockefeller Foundation. He played a crucial role in improving the health and sanitation of a fellow South-East Asian country, the Philippines. Working there from 1903 to 1915 as first its Chief Quarantine Officer and then later, its Director of Health, he ran an exhaustive programme to eradicate cholera, plague, smallpox, hookworm, leprosy, yaws and malaria in the country. Were David's intentions for coming to Singapore similar? Was it the fulfilment of Rudyard Kipling's '*White Man's Burden*'?

He brushes off the insinuation with disinterest. "I'm a child of an immigrant family. I didn't have any burden." It was, to him, an opportunity to travel to somewhere tropical and exotic, where history was in the process of being made. It was not with the intention of making history in Singapore. "I came partly because I grew up during the Vietnam conflict, and I had never been educated about Asia. I learned a little bit of Western European history in school and university, but very little about Asia. I read '*Fire in the Lake*' about the history of Vietnam, and was fascinated. I knew about Sukarno, followed by Suharto, and the issues there and the killings. I was fascinated. Singapore was a first world place to come and be immediately adjacent to third world issues, and I thought, '*This is the best thing ever!*'"

How did a young, white guy from Texas, with a full head of hair, end up on this sunny island?

"This would have been 1988 [when he was between the ages of 30–31]. I was the Chief Resident doing some research work still at Rockefeller University, on top of clinical work." He had been involved in two projects at Rockefeller — identifying anti-oncogenes using a Wilm's tumour model, and bioengineering anti-sense RNA to suppress HIV replication *in vitro*. "I was about to become a faculty member, essentially one year out from my training. And I was asked to come to Singapore to give a talk about infections in immunocompromised hosts." David was the Chief Resident of Medicine, traditionally performed after Fellowship in the Cornell programme, from 1988 to 1989. This was a valuable, sought after, post-Fellowship position which typically led to a faculty position. This was a position that Dr Anthony Fauci himself helmed between 1971 and 1972.

But first, we got him to pause there and took a few steps back. How did such an opportunity even land on his lap, considering that he would have just been a young upstart?

"When I was an Internal Medicine trainee, from 1984 to 1986, a group of Singaporean doctors in training appeared in my hospital in New York [New York Hospital] to further their careers. These were Wong Meng Chong, a Neurologist, Ngoi Sing Shang, a Colorectal Surgeon, and John Wong Eu Li, an Internist and then Haematologist/Oncologist. They introduced Singapore as a possible destination to me..." He deliberates for a moment before continuing. "And probably placed my name in the ear of MOH decision makers as the person to pilot ID in Singapore."

We spoke to Prof John Wong, who had been there right from the very beginning. He had been an intern in New York Hospital, in 1985, when he first met David, who was then an Assistant Chief Resident beginning his final year of Internal Medicine residency. During David's ID Fellowship from 1986 to 1988, Prof Wong did indeed try to persuade David to consider Singapore as a place to further his career. Amongst the many ID physicians he had conversed with, David was the only one who was willing to take a stab in the dark to come to Singapore.[22]

David continued, painting his side of the story on why his services were sought after. "Singapore was interested because the Permanent Secretary for Health at the time was a Haematologist, one of the first Haematologists ever trained here or trained at all. His name was Kwa Soon Bee. He's also the architect of the modern healthcare system in Singapore to a certain degree, with an emphasis on specialist medicine and advanced medical care in Singapore. He saw where Medicine was. He was a well-informed leader. He had advisors who were seeing problems on the ground with immunocompromised hosts, and the limitations of the existing capacity to support their care. Feng Pao Hsii was a Rheumatologist, giving cyclosporine and steroids as part of his practice, and observing both the benefit and potential for harm with immunosuppression. He knew additional professional support was needed. He was one of the impetuses for Infectious Diseases developing as a specialty. He had spent time overseas, saw how Infectious Diseases supported clinical care, and realised the benefit ID could be to Singapore. Singapore was going to have more immunocompromised patients — cancer treatment and organ transplant programmes, in particular kidney transplants, had begun not for very long. And they were running into problems with opportunistic infections. Some patients were dying."

Up till then, Infectious Diseases had not been a recognised specialty in Singapore. Communicable diseases were rife in the city state during the pre- and post-independence era, and beyond certain conditions such as tuberculosis and sexually transmitted infections which were managed in specialist clinics, general practitioners, physicians, and surgeons handled common infections regularly in their daily practice. Those with communicable diseases such as cholera or smallpox were managed at Middleton Hospital, or what was subsequently known as the Communicable Disease Centre (CDC) at Moulmein Road, and these were on the wane. What was becoming complicated and problematic at that point in time was the management of hospital-based infectious diseases, grappling with immunocompromised patients and their innumerable infections, as well as rapidly evolving antimicrobial resistance. Clinical Microbiologists were on hand to provide specialist input if needed, but they were already mired deep in laboratory duties, and direct patient care could not be provided optimally.

"Kwa Soon Bee and Feng Pao Hsii realised there was a problem. And Clinical Microbiology at that time was not really designed to handle them. They were overwhelmed with work where they were — in the laboratory. And immunocompromised hosts were not a particular focus at that time."

Without the late Prof Kwa Soon Bee or Prof Feng Pao Hsii around to share their side of the story, we turned to Prof Chee Yam Cheng, who corroborated this story for us.[23] Sometime back in the 1980s, Prof Feng Pao Hsii had sought his help, in his capacity as the Director of Medical Manpower at MOH at that time, in bringing ID specialists to Singapore. The crux of it all was that Prof Feng's lupus patients were getting esoteric infections. Somewhere in that time frame, HIV had also been discovered and was becoming a threat (the first case of HIV was admitted to the CDC in 1985), so the impetus for ID specialists was greatly supported. As had been done with the Geriatric specialty, the same formula for starting a new specialty service was pursued. This involved getting a good overseas specialist prepared to spend 5 or more years in Singapore to train local doctors, before sending the latter overseas for HMDP.[24] Eventually, they would return to be staff of the department. With that model, Prof Feng sought advice from his good friends in the University of California, San Francisco, for names as well as conferences in the US to attend, so that he could speak to these specialists. Eventually, Prof Feng concluded that David was a suitable candidate, and they got him employed under MOH to work with Prof Feng at TTSH,[25] as well as to help run Middleton Hospital. To be clear, David denies having met Prof Feng until he formally arrived in Singapore in 1989 and was placed in his department.

It was, therefore, still a bit of a mystery to us as to how David's name surfaced to MOH, but Prof John Wong was there to help connect the dots.[22] Prof Wong's father, the late Dr Wong Heck Sing, who was then the Deputy Chairman of the Public Service Commission (PSC), had heard from his son about David, and was also privy to the need for an ID service in Singapore to bolster the medical community. Back then, the PSC was in charge of interviewing and hiring consultants for the public health sector. Dr Wong had also been friends with the late Prof Kwa Soon Bee, and it was apparently he who suggested to Prof Kwa that David, with his stellar credentials, could be considered to help lay the foundations of ID here in Singapore.

But before all that, David was required to prove his worth and commitment. "I was invited to come from New York in 1988 to give a series of Grand Rounds on opportunistic infections in immunocompromised hosts and general infectious diseases. Unbeknownst to me, the invitation to speak was a preamble to assess if and how ID, and me, might be useful if a longer term stay in Singapore was offered. I was put up on the top floor of SGH[26] Block 6, in one of several 1-bedroom, utilitarian, over-air conditioned, damp, under-lit, smelling of disinfectant and burning mosquito coil, kitchen-less, efficiency flats they had at that time." This, though, did not put him off. "I was smitten." We weren't quite sure if 'smothered' was what he actually meant. But we carry on.

"I attended morning hospital rounds at least once with a SGH medical unit on that visit. I cannot recall which team or the consultants who led rounds. I was surprised that rounds routinely began at 8 AM — I was accustomed to 7 AM. The rounds I attended were also notable for their anecdotal, non-literature-based, didactic quality. Decision making and plans were not so much discussed as dictated. It was a new experience for me." It was more likely a rude awakening.

He adds. "I was amazed when I came to speak. It was at the College of Medicine building on the campus at SGH. I gave several talks, but one of the talks was on a Sunday afternoon, in a large lecture hall. It was not air-conditioned, but fans were on. And the room was packed. There had to be 100 to 200 people, and I thought, '*What the hell is wrong with these people that they would come to a talk on a Sunday afternoon? Is there nothing on TV? Why aren't they at home or playing golf or doing something else instead of listening to some guy talk?*'" There was truth behind the satire — we were, and still are, a nation of workaholics, and one of the most overworked countries in the world.[27]

"I gave the series of talks, was probed whether I might be interested in a job here, then went back to the States. And then I received a letter from Chee Yam Cheng, who was in charge of recruiting, HMDP awarding, and a variety of things. He had a thousand jobs. He's capable of handling many more. The letter was out of the blue, this terse note saying, in so many words, '*You are instructed to come to Singapore.*'"

At this point, he looks at us with his characteristic twinkle in the eyes and cheeky grin, seemingly like it was just yesterday that he had received the call up. And he answered it like a good Singaporean son would, without missing a beat. "And I was like, '*Cool! I have no idea how this is going to go. I'm going to do that.*'"

Here we see a trademark of David's — fearlessness or foolhardiness you may call it, two sides of the same coin. A young man, full of self-confidence, a hint of a swagger, willing to give up a burgeoning career in the States to come to this academic backwater of an island on a whim. How did the senior members of his faculty take to the news?

"By the time the letter arrived, I was a young faculty guy, in a moderate-sized department. I was told, '*You'll be Assistant Professor for X number of years. An Associate Professor of X number of years, a full Professor after that. You'll vacation with us on Shelter Island and then you'll die. That's your life.*' And I was like, '*Wow, okay, that's reassuring.*'"

David's reply was mordacious — he clearly wasn't sold.

"My Head of the Medicine department told me not to go. It would be the death of my career. The Infectious Diseases fraternity is small; you'll be seen as someone who doesn't follow orders and doing it '*the way*' it's supposed to be done." He emphasises '*the way*' with air quotes.

"He said, '*If we want you to go to Singapore, we'll send you to Singapore.*' He had been President of the IDSA. He was like the Godfather." He brings up the iconic fictional gangster of the '70s, Vito Corleone, made famous in the film, '*The Godfather*'. An offer by him was something one simply could not refuse.

"If the Head of Medicine said '*Don't do it*', you don't do it. Anyway, that was the feeling, and the feeling was that this wasn't the right way. They weren't being possessive. They were just stating the facts, '*What you're proposing isn't the right way to go about doing it.*'"

Thus, in October 1989, unwilling to be stifled by local authority, David decided to exchange it for the stifling heat of the tropical climate altogether. And ironically, in Singapore, not exactly a place renowned for libertarian values.

"I had decided I didn't want to grow old in the States, so it was an easy decision for me."

It couldn't have been that easy a decision altogether, surely. After all, he'd be unsupported here. He'd have none of the intellectual support from more experienced peers and colleagues that he could bounce ideas off. And this was in the pre-internet and pre-Google era. Memory correlated more with the amount of grey matter one had between the ears, rather than the number of bytes one had on hand.

"It was similar to jumping out of an airplane. It was exciting. It really was. I was in a flop sweat for the first few months. You're just in a constant sweat going, '*Oh my god!*' Weight loss. I didn't sleep. It was very stressful, but incredibly rewarding professionally."

"You know why? You're in a position that you can harm people, and you're given the luxury of trust to 'succeed or fail'. If you do something wrong…" His voice trails off at this point, realising the burden of responsibility that he had carried in those early years. "People are depending on you." Colleagues. Peers. Friends. Patients. *Primum non nocere.*

So who or what could he rely on?

"The library at NUS, the medical library, was pretty good. It was open till 1 or 2 AM, so I would round, get there by eight and stay there till midnight. I was reading journals that were a few months behind, but good enough because I came from a journal-based world when I was in New York. I mean, my US experience was all literature-based, so it was thrilling to have access to familiar journals in Singapore. And my fund of knowledge came from my extensive clinical experience in New York as well as reading and memorizing '*Principles and Practice of ID*' from stem to stern in preparation for my exit exams, so I felt pretty good about my breadth. It was more the depth that I lacked. And Singapore helped me to fill it in. It helped me quickly fill in the cracks, plus what I could glean from the literature. Having access to the medical library was equivalent to having a security blanket — I was comforted and confident."

It would seem that he had benefited from being in Singapore as much as Singapore had benefited from him being here. In nature, 'symbiosis' describes this mutually beneficial relationship aptly.

At this juncture, we enquired about something even more fundamental. As a multi-cultural and still relatively young nation, a significant proportion of the population would still be conversing in their mother tongue, be it Mandarin, and its multitude of dialects, or Malay, or Tamil. The 'Speak Good English Movement' was not formally launched until the year 2000 by then Prime Minister Goh Chok Tong. It was used to combat the rise of our very own English dialect, Singlish, a hodgepodge of all the languages spoken in this city-state, so that we could be ready to take on the rest of the world. Was he not concerned about the potential language barrier?

"I had already moved from Texas to New York, and that was a bit of a linguistic challenge for me. The colloquial English spoken in the US northeast was distinct from that spoken in Texas. I had to learn the patois. Coming to Singapore was not really dramatically different. The way people speak can sometimes sound a little choppy to my ear when I was younger, but I would say, within a week, I felt reasonably comfortable. Now, what shocked me in 1989, and still shocks me today, is the number of acronyms used. Often gratuitously. The institutionalized use of acronyms and the potential for miscommunication remains troubling to this day. Getting back to your point, I had to learn to understand Singlish. But I had Mun San, Sin Yew and Yee-Sin to help me out." These would be the pioneer batch of ID trainees in Singapore — Dr Lam Mun San, Dr Wong Sin Yew, and Prof Leo Yee-Sin.

A legend had also been propagated through the years that David, upon his arrival in Singapore, was treated like a hippie because he had long hair. They, the hippies, were associated with drugs and permissive and deviant behaviour, and back in the early '70s, the Singapore government launched Operation Snip Snip, whereby men with long hair were required to get a haircut before being allowed into Singapore.[28] Was it true that David had to have his locks chopped off before being allowed through immigration?

He baits us by obfuscating. "Long hair was the fashion in West Texas and in my social circles during the era of my teens and twenties. I was not an adherent of the hippie subculture. My hair was relatively short by the time I arrived in Singapore. By the mid-1990s it had grown out again, but my thinning pate eventually made that coiffure less a fashion statement and more a wistful holdout; thus, it was shorn..."

He leaves us hanging for a moment.

"However, not in Changi Airport."

And the rumour gets quashed.

We returned back to the topic. So how does one single Infectious Diseases physician systemically go about colonising the healthcare system?

"You first establish that what you can provide is of added value. You determine who the various stakeholders are, who has an interest in participating in the grand experiment. And you need to understand what they think you are there to do. When I came to Singapore, it was trying to figure out who were the players that were interested in Infectious Diseases succeeding, and who might be threatened by Infectious Diseases. Have conversations with them and try to see if I could indeed help their patients and ease their burden."

At this point, a recurring theme of relevance starts to appear. His need to be, and to remain, relevant, resonates throughout the interview. "And the specialty of Infectious Diseases could be of value to them. I was convinced it could. But I had to understand first the culture of what is valued. When I came here, in most of the teaching institutions, knowing the latest literature was not necessarily valued. I had to understand what was valued and that allowed me to angle the pitch, to be able to meet their needs."

And who was this *them* that he sought approval from?

"The first group included those who wanted to see Infectious Diseases succeed, and those who may want to see it to fail."

We wondered if the Clinical Microbiologists of the day belonged in that latter category. Did they feel threatened by his presence? For this, we sought to find out more from the current head of the National Public Health Laboratory, Prof Raymond Lin.[29] He had been a Microbiology trainee back when David first arrived, and he attests that the development of the ID specialty was supported by the chief Microbiologist back then, Dr Jimmy Sng. It had been a natural and much needed development — there were not enough Clinical Microbiologists to fulfil that clinical role, and to do it in a sustainable way. No loss was perceived, and in fact, David was found to be a good bridge between the Clinical Microbiologists and the newly-formed ID specialty. He, Prof Lin, had regularly been invited to participate in the very same clinical rounds conducted by David that was attended by the first batch of ID trainees, one of whom included Prof Leo Yee-Sin. Prof Leo herself would go on to front ID in Singapore, becoming the Executive Director of Singapore's National Centre for Infectious Diseases (NCID) between 2017 and 2023. This relationship between the two specialties, fostered at the beginning and nurtured by David over the years, paid dividends down the road, when the two specialties had to, and are still continuing to, work in tandem to handle infectious diseases crises that afflict Singapore.

David continues. "The second group extended beyond that, proselytizing into the greater medical community and into the non-medical community to educate. Because that's one of the roles we do as ID physicians — community education. So conceptually, that was the strategy."

"In order to proselytize, I gave lots of talks, and back then, I had many slide decks. I went around with four or five carousels of slides in my car on any given day. I'd sit outside one of the hospitals in my car between rounds and talks to produce a lecture from the slides available. I'd start off in the morning at one hospital, give a talk, then see patients. Then I'd sit outside another hospital, reconfiguring the slides to give the next talk. I had hundreds, if not thousands of slides, and I knew every one of them intimately, and could reorder them pretty quickly."

Following this advertising blitz and marketing his wares, he had to now walk the talk.

"Because I didn't know everybody, because I was starting anew, the one thing I knew how to do was be a good Infectious Diseases physician. So, I went about being a good Infectious Diseases physician. I went about asking others to allow me to demonstrate what Infectious Diseases could offer them. And then do it by hard work, by example. Getting my trainees to understand that ID consultation and management was not just '*How long do I give the antibiotic for*', but to educate and to show there's methodology to this. It isn't just a brainstem reflex. There are concepts to guide us. There's proper application."

"So, we did that and interest in our work grew by word of mouth. It spread quickly that what we were doing helped, and that we're not here to interfere with anybody's workflow. If anything, we were here to help their workflow. Everybody, as always in a public health institution, has a large volume of work to complete in a given day. Any way you can help them get it done results in you becoming their friend. You're going to make their day a bit better. That was a way to ingratiate Infectious Diseases into the medical community quickly."

Prof Brenda Ang, who had then just returned from her ID training at the Mayo Clinic, admits that, depending on the persons and the departments, there were mixed reactions to David's arrival.[30] He started by seeing referrals for interesting and difficult infections, and was thus much appreciated in SGH by the Burns Department, the Renal Department especially for transplant, and the Cardiothoracic Department, which had been about to start heart transplant services. The more senior staff in the medical departments could not quite place him, and thought he was not doing the job he was assigned to do. He was, after all, in a General Medical (GM) department, but did not want to run a GM ward, or do the usual GM duties, which was understandable, as he was much more in demand for seeing the difficult infections in ICUs, Burns, and Haematology. And he was also getting referrals from a few other different hospitals.

David knew he came in as an outsider, and consciously sought to foster relationships, making himself relatable. "Being a non-judgemental friend, I wasn't there to take their job. I'm not trying to be arrogant. I'm not trying to know it all. I'm a struggling academic like everyone else. Trying to do a good job. We all, whether you're in the United States or Europe or Singapore, struggle daily. Let's embrace that. Let's share that beauty and privilege of practicing Medicine, that art of Medicine. It's imperfect."

It's hard to imagine him breaking out in a sweat, let alone struggling, with the tasks at hand. Especially when he appeared so nonchalant just moments ago about jumping into the abyss. How did he go about building his team?

"I came in October 1989 as an employee of MOH. I was initially with Rheumatology and Internal Medicine in Medical Unit IV, which was the home of TTSH's Rheumatology and Clinical Immunology community, and then one ID physician. I was answerable, interestingly enough, to the Rheumatologist, Prof Feng Pao Hsii, and his division. Because he was most interested in Infectious Diseases. And my litter mates in the department included Chng Hiok Hee, Howe Hwee Siew and Boey Mee Leng."

And here, he digresses a bit to speak about typical Singaporean traits he first encountered there. "These are strong, capable, independent thinking people. They could be quite fierce, but they were kind to me. Feng

Pao Hsii was a master at handling us all. And he was, to be honest with you, well-travelled and comfortable in all worlds. So, I assume he volunteered to have me join his unit as he could be the cultural translator, the intellectual sparring partner, as well as the icebreaker, to prevent me from upsetting people I shouldn't alienate. He was a master at understanding how the system worked. He knew MOH, he knew what was expected of ID. He knew how to get things done. He was quite good at telling me, '*Wait, don't waste your time approaching the problem the way you're planning. You'll get nowhere. Go talk to this person.*' He was the first president of the SIDS.[31] He was a very good man."

SIDS had been set up, in 1990, by Prof Feng Pao Hsii and a group of like-minded doctors with an interest in the advancement of ID in Singapore. David had just formally arrived in Singapore a few months back, and was one of the founding members of the society. Physicians with an interest in ID, as well as Clinical Microbiologists, would make up the rest of the group. According to the minutes of the inaugural meeting, Prof Feng felt that there was '*sustained momentum in the development of this discipline locally*', and decided that it was timely to have this society '*formed to maintain this interest*'. This was one of the foundational blocks in getting ID integrated as a mainstream specialty, which would only happen in 1998, when the specialist accreditation board for ID was finally approved.

We return back to David, who was finding his feet in a new world. He shared with us his daily duties.

"I taught and provided inpatient clinical support and rotary clinic outpatient support ad hoc in TTSH, but would go to CDC to provide inpatient care to those with AIDS in Ward 76. Having been trained and on staff in New York City in the 1980s, I had extensive experience managing persons living with AIDS, and Dr Monteiro was eager to work together."

This would have been Dr Edmund Monteiro, the son of Dr Ernest Stevens Monteiro of polio vaccine fame. The older Monteiro had been the medical superintendent of Middleton Hospital, which had been renamed as "伝染病院" (Densen Byoin, or 'Infectious Disease Hospital' in Japanese), during the Japanese Occupation, and the younger Monteiro grew up on the grounds of the hospital. He later joined the hospital in 1965, before following in his father's footsteps to become its medical director in 1980. David fondly recounts his experiences with the younger Monteiro, who could be said to be one of the pioneers of ID in Singapore.

"Dr Monteiro is a generous soul. He had grown up on the grounds of CDC when his father was the Medical Superintendent. As such, Dr Monteiro knew everyone who worked there and often their families — from the sweeper to the Sister [senior nurse]. He was gracious with the staff and had a heart of service for patients. He was fatherly, empathetic and could be appropriately stern with naughty patients when needed. His bedside manner recalled the old-school family doctor of my youth — not in a hurry, wanting to hear what you had to say, eager to help your condition and the reasons for your condition. The pace of work in CDC in the 1980s and early '90s provided the opportunity to deliver less rushed individual care — inpatient volume was not huge. That said, he had mastered his domain of communicable disease, by decades of experience and pragmatism. He shared clinical pearls gleaned from his years of service which were often not in textbooks, and he played a major role in the ID trainee's communicable diseases education."

Business soon became brisk. "I quickly spread out from TTSH because Kwa Soon Bee, who was the Permanent Secretary for Health, would call me into the office every once in a while, and ask, *'How's it going?'* And one day he said, *'You need to be in SGH.'* I do not recall if it was 1990 or '91."

Once over at SGH, resistance and precedence were overcome with charm and a bit of guile. "When I initially started seeing patients, they [the physicians] were going, *'We know how to prescribe antibiotics, infectious diseases are over at CDC. That's where malaria and cholera go to be cared for.'* Then I responded with, *'But I can help you treat this guy with endocarditis with less toxicity, relapse and cost.'* They said *'We're doing what Prof wants us to do.'* Without breaking anybody's rice bowl, I had to show the value of ID. I had to prove it in a non-threatening way, and show that nobody's ego was going to be bruised. I'm just trying to make everybody's job a little easier and improve patient outcomes."

The last piece of the tertiary hospital puzzle was NUH. "Tan Yew Oo, who was the Head of Medicine and a Haematologist, asked that I see his immunocompromised patients in NUH. They weren't doing stem cell transplants then, but they were treating leukaemics and similarly vulnerable patients. Prof Tan had trained in Canada, where he had experience using ID services."

Interestingly enough, David isn't the first Infectious Diseases specialist in Singapore. "There was a physician at NUH who had trained in Infectious Diseases in Canada as well, Prof Ti Teow-Yee. She returned to Singapore before I arrived. When she came back, the Singapore Medical Council (SMC) did not recognise her formal training in Canada, as there was not an ID division at that time, so she worked out of the Department of Pharmacology."

We pause here to take stock of the situation. In 1989, the year that David arrived in Singapore, Dr Edmund Monteiro was managing communicable diseases over at the CDC. Prof Ti Teow-Yee had been trained in ID in Canada, and was practicing in NUH whilst also seeing referrals at SGH once a week; her ID training though had not been recognised locally. Prof Helen Oh was the first physician sent for HMDP (ID) to the University of British Columbia, Vancouver, in 1989; and Prof Brenda Ang would soon follow suit, training in ID at the Mayo Clinic in Rochester, Minnesota, in the United States, from 1990 to 1992. Prof Leo Yee-Sin, Dr Wong Sin Yew, and Dr Lam Mun San joined David as his registrars not too long after his arrival in 1989. We proceeded to ask a leading question at this juncture — why had he been able to successfully plant the ID flag in Singapore whilst those before him had only been met with frustration?

He cites three major factors. "Those ID physicians before me had pre-defined key performance indicators which did not include ID work. Also, there was non-recognition of the speciality, and there were pre-existing mindsets to counter." He was cognizant of the fact that he did not have that many hoops to jump through. "I had only the last item to contend with as I was brought on specifically to do ID."

Like our forefathers who had first arrived in Singapore from overseas and took root, David presided over a rapidly expanding Infectious Diseases family.

"Chee Yam Cheng either identified or solicited trainees who might have an interest in Infectious Diseases. I don't think they, the early trainees, were conscripted to ID. I think it was volitional. I did nothing to recruit other than appear, and then I was introduced to these three registrars immediately. Then Helen and Brenda came back from their training abroad and joined us. So, I don't know if they'd been naughty and this was some sort of punishment, but I don't think so. No, I think they were all saying, '*This sounds interesting.*' Credit all goes to them for saying, '*Some guy, comes from a different country, whom we don't know, whose educational background we don't know, is going to lead this effort.*' The credit goes to them for jumping out of the airplane and agreeing to work with me."

"I spread them out because the demand had grown by the time Brenda and Helen had come back. Brenda and Sin Yew went to SGH. Yee-Sin and Mun San were primarily at TTSH. And Helen made her way to Changi [General Hospital]. I would convene, what became Grand Ward rounds, with them weekly. I drove around to every hospital, conversed with them regularly to make sure they were supported. We didn't have a SMC-recognised training programme set up at that time. That said, the training was two years with me, and then a year or more on HMDP, and that was it. There was no exit exam. Yee-Sin, Mun San and Sin Yew were sent off for HMDPs after they'd been with me for a couple of years. But I would tell you, their workload while in Singapore was substantial. When they were gone on HMDP, those of us still here worked hard. That was a breather for them [those who had gone on HMDP]. Ha!"

His original intention for ID in Singapore was that of a hub-and-spoke model. The specialists and trainees would have a base in CDC from which to venture out to the various public healthcare institutions (PHI) to render services. At least at the beginning. "It was a means to ensure the trainees developed a bedrock of ID expertise before being distracted by the work exigencies other than ID that exist in the other PHIs." He felt that this was the most feasible model at that time, but knew that ultimately, each individual hospital would go on to set up its own independent ID divisions. "I knew that would occur. My thinking was to set a standard of excellence first, then let a thousand blossoms bloom."

We took a left turn here. We were flummoxed — was this a deliberate misquotation of Mao Zedong, the leader and founder of the People's

Republic of China? In Mao's Hundred Flowers Campaign in 1956, he coined the expression, '百花齐放，百家争鸣' [bǎi huā qí fàng, bǎi jiā zhēng míng], '*Let a hundred flowers bloom; let a hundred schools of thought contend*'. Under the guise of seeking the opinions and suggestions of China's intellectuals, and even allowing for criticism of the party and its policies, Mao then subsequently targeted these same dissidents in the Anti-Rightist campaign in 1957, rounding them up by the hundreds of thousands and shipping them off for execution or re-education[32]. David reassures us that he was, instead, misquoting George H. W. Bush, the 41st President of the United States, in his acceptance speech at the Republican presidential nomination in 1988. In it, he made a pledge to the nation to '*keep America moving forward, always forward, for a better America, for an endless enduring dream and a thousand points of light.*' David acknowledges his 'error', as always, with humour. "I've mangled and stolen the quote from multiple sources!" We 'reassured' him that we, too, couldn't promise not to mangle his quotes in future.

And where does Prof Paul Tambyah factor in? We knew Prof Tambyah was the first Division Head of Infectious Diseases in NUH where we were currently practicing, and we were curious to know if David had a hand in this.

"He was an MO then. I knew of his dad who had asked me to see a couple of patients in Mount Elizabeth Hospital. And Paul, he looked no different back then, except he had a little more hair. He asked me if I would write a reference letter for him to use in applying for US training. As a young faculty member involved in screening applicants for training in New York, I'd received many flowery letters regarding candidates from far flung countries without basis for interpreting the letters. There was coded language used by US faculty writing letters for their own candidates that overseas letter writers did not use. If a Singaporean mentor wrote a letter to the States at that time in support of an applicant from Singapore, the response from the receiving institution may have been, '*Where the hell is Singapore? What part of China is Singapore?*' I'd been involved in US medical education, and in bringing people from all over the United States to New York Hospital to speak and to be involved in our education programme — I knew people all around the US. I could write to them and say, '*Look, I've either invited your Head or I've invited you to come speak, and I'm legitimate. Here's my* bona fides. *Let me just get a foot in the door. Please take this person and I promise you he or she will cost you no money, and you'll see him or her to be of value.*' Paul wanted to go to Chicago, so I wrote a letter there, and he got in. He always teases me, saying half the letter was about me. But the problem was, I had to introduce myself to them and use the coded language to establish credibility. Paul tells me he was just a passing reference in this arrangement."

"'*It worked, didn't it? You got in!*'" He jests back, tongue-in-cheek. In the real world, he has nothing but the utmost respect for Prof Tambyah, although he doesn't occasionally mind taking the mickey out of him.

We cornered Prof Tambyah on this and he sought to clarify one aspect, that the letter David wrote for him was not enough to get into RUSH Medical College. Instead, he 'only' got into an 'Ellis Island' programme at Weiss Memorial, which was then under the University of Chicago, for his Internal Medicine training.[33] 'Ellis Island' hospitals supposedly cared for the marginalized populations in the States, and residents feared training in them, as compared to 'Mayflower' hospitals, which cared for the rest.

It was, ultimately, all just a bit of an ongoing banter.

Prof Chong Chia Yin, one of the pioneers of Paediatric Infectious Diseases in Singapore, and currently a senior consultant at KK Women's and Children's Hospital (KKH), shared with us too that David was instrumental in helping Paediatric ID get set up in Singapore.[34] Prior to the new KKH opening in 1997, TTSH and SGH both had their own individual paediatric units. These eventually became parked under the Children's hospital portion, together with the existing KKH neonatal unit, in KKH in 1997. Prof Chong, who was initially based at TTSH, started out seeing paediatric as well as adult ID cases together with David in 1993. She had found him to be extremely knowledgeable, but what made an even deeper impression on her was the amount of time and effort he made to keep updated, as well as his collegiality with his colleagues.

But establishing an Infectious Diseases service from scratch is not like having a blank canvas to paint a masterpiece, but rather, firefighting on multiple fronts. Beyond providing clinical services nationwide and indoctrinating his registrars, his role as an Infectious Diseases physician would encompass, non-exhaustively, proffering other services such as Infection Prevention and Control and Antimicrobial Stewardship. How did he tackle being swamped on so many different fronts?

"You had to prioritise. What is the most important thing? Why am I here? What can Infectious Diseases do to endear itself, to ingratiate itself, to integrate itself, and establish itself such that *we can't live without it now*. I had to do that first, which was clinical work and easing everybody's burden."

"When we get into things like Antibiotic Stewardship and Infection Prevention and Control, there was a certain amount of *'don't want to know, full stop'*, or, *'don't want to know because the solution is painful'*. It's going to cost money. It's going to cost manpower. We're not ready for that yet."

You could sense, here, that even the boundless enthusiasm and energy of youth could be worn down by endless bureaucracy.

"I had to be able to address Quality Assurance topics in a way that was acceptable. I could either express frustration, or say, *'No, if we fix this, it'll fix a whole host of other problems.'* Because the energy of activation to solve this problem was so much, it didn't matter that it saved an enormous amount down the road. The commitment of time, human resources and funding was just too much now. I understood that. I had no problems with it. It was frustrating because I thought we should invest in a tonne of Infectious Diseases training and expand quickly. We could get many people trained, but it wasn't a priority at the time. I thought we should be doing clinical research, basic research. Neither were priorities at that time. So, it's okay. I understood."

It seems that he is still trying to come to terms with this fact even now, after all these years. Providing health to the general population was immensely more complicated than providing healthcare down on the ground.

"Singapore had and has finite resources, the government has services it needs to provide, leaders have to decide at any point in time how to best allocate those resources." And so the approach was to tackle the myriad problems piecemeal, whilst continuing to prove his and the specialty's worth.

"We'll get a part-time infection prevention nurse. And then do selected projects. And we'll see how it goes. The trick was, show the decision makers that this saves lives, saves money, and saves resources. Then, if you invest a little bit more, we can do even more."

We took a break from clinical duties to hear about some of the side hustles David had been engaged in during his first Singapore stint. He had two incidents that he had been itching to tell us, both of which, unsurprisingly, did not stray far from the topic of infectious diseases.

"It would have been between '92–93. I was rounding at SGH, and I was asked to see a professional hunter warded there, who had come from an island off the coast of Sumbawa — Moyo Island. He had moderate parasite load *Plasmodium vivax* [a species of *Plasmodium*, a parasite that caused malaria]. He was a big Caucasian dude from South Africa, and he had a huge defect in his leg from an old injury, when a boar had stabbed him with its tusk. He was really sick with malaria. Anyway, he responded to therapy and was discharged, and it turns out that he was employed by Adrian Zecha as a hunting guide at Amanwana [then a new luxury resort on Moyo Island]."

"Adrian Zecha was an Indonesian of Dutch and Chinese descent. He became involved in the hospitality business and opened Amanwana. He had hired this gentleman [the patient with malaria] to take hotel guests hunting. The island is pretty big. They had some, I think, deer, but I don't think there were rhinos. I forget what they were hunting. Anyway, he acquired malaria at the resort during its soft opening. Quite a number of workers and villagers on the island were found to be infected as well."

"He [the guide] improved, went back, and then the next thing I know, I get a call saying, '*Look, we've got a problem on the island with a lot of people. We had a soft opening, but we can't have our guests getting malaria. Can you come help us out?*' An entourage led by Adrian, including his friends and guests, and me, flew to Sumbawa, then took a speedboat to Moyo."

"We treated all the infected, including radical cures with primaquine [an anti-malarial drug] to all we could find in the villages. I didn't personally treat each individual; I had a contracted nurse licensed to practice in Indonesia who was seconded to Amanwana, and we came up with the strategy. She acquired chloroquine and primaquine, arranged for patient education, drug distribution, rudimentary adherence assurance, and subsequent monitoring. It was a very rewarding experience. There continued to be sporadic cases of malaria due to travel, but our intervention dramatically decreased the numbers. Amanwana went through their opening successfully."

"Because of that good deed, when I subsequently passed through Sumbawa, I was invited to stay at Amanwana. While backpacking through the Indonesian archipelago in 1994, I stayed for a week to recuperate from my travels. It was wonderful."

It was an incredible story, and made even incredibly more so when we chanced upon an article about this incident, published by the South China Morning Post in 1993.[35] This was a resort that even the then Princess of Wales, Princess Diana, had graced. The story goes that guests and employees at the resort were coming down with malaria, and both business and reputation had taken a hit as a result of this unwanted guest. It subsequently eradicated the disease with '*experts, like the head of the communicable diseases centre in Singapore, [who had] come in to help us.*' That would have been David, even though he was not mentioned by name. We were gobsmacked, and so was he.

He was quick to qualify. "I was unaware of the article until you brought it to my attention! To my recollection, I was not representing Singapore, Singapore MOH, or CDC, on my trip to Moyo."

The next tale was a favourite of ours, and clearly one of his as well. Veterinarians, if you have any as friends, frequently like to emphasise the point that they have a broader set of skills, having to deal with a variety of species, as compared to medical doctors, who only have to deal with one. One thing for certain is that bacteria, and all other pathogens, are agnostic as to whom or what they infect. David too was mostly agnostic to those who sought his expertise, and his distinctive skillsets were called upon from an unlikely source.

"This was probably in 1990 or 1991. I received a call from Shirley Yeo, a Singaporean who had trained in the US as a big-animal veterinarian.

She, I believe, had already interned or worked at a zoo in the US, and was recruited back to Singapore to be the chief veterinarian for the Singapore Zoo. We were both quite young at the time."

"She called me up and said, '*Look, I have this clinic here [in the Singapore Zoo] and it's pretty awesome. From a surgical perspective, I couldn't ask for more. But I've drugs in my pharmacy that I'm not sure how best to use.*' So I went specifically to help with the antibiotics. She had everything — quinolones, aminoglycosides, cephalosporins [different classes of antibiotics] — it was spectacular what she had available."

"She said, '*I need you to help me.*' I said, '*Well, I know nothing about reptiles or birds, which are reptiles.*'" He was alluding to the fact that birds are the evolutionary descendants of dinosaurs, which were reptiles.[36] "'*I can probably deal with your mammals to a degree. You'll have to figure out doses, and you'll have to tell me what you think is wrong with them.*' She had access, I think, to the SGH lab at the time." As always, he could never say no, and with that, he became a visiting ID veterinarian consultant to the Singapore Zoological Gardens, as it was known back then.

We did some investigative work and managed to track down Dr Shirley Yeo Llizo, who was now the Director of Animal Health at the Topeka Zoo and Conservation Centre in Kansas, US. She did not recall how she came to know of David 30 years ago, though she vividly remembers their first encounter one late afternoon, where he was standing by the entrance to the zoo hospital. He wore glasses, and had longish, wavy hair. She was quick to emphasise, though, that it was still above the collar.[37]

David brought us round to his first consult — it was a paediatric case. "The first patient she called me up for was a baby orangutan with pox lesions. I went out and saw the baby orangutan, which was being held by the mother. It was in the evening because I got out there after work. And while I was waiting to see my paediatric patient, because we had to have the zookeepers around for me to safely attend to the patient, you could see all the orangutans returning to their bunkhouse to settle in for the night. They would grab a burlap sack, and they have bunk beds, and you can see the mothers with the babies going in first. They grab a burlap sack, which is their bedding, and go find their bunk for the night. And then you'd see the adult males going in, and they are…not sombre but very quiet, sort of going about their ways. And then you'd see the teenage orangutans. And they're rowdy. It was fascinating to observe their lives 'behind the scenes.'"

"Anyway, I saw the afflicted baby while she was being held by her mother, and found the vesicles on her haunch. I scraped the vesicles to do a Tzanck prep." The Tzanck smear, described by the French physician Arnault Tzanck in 1947, is one of the quick investigative tests performed to detect the presence of herpesvirus infections. "Scraping orangutan skin is different than human. So that was weird." Dr Yeo gives her input at this juncture, explaining that the skin on their limbs was more pliable than humans, felt thin but was not really so, and had a tacky feel almost like an old person's skin.

Was he wearing any personal protective equipment?

"No, no, no, only gloves."

We were aghast. Speak to an Infectious Diseases physician and any symptom or sign, any pet or pest, could be linked with a particular pathogen, and sometimes even more than one. Vesicular lesions on the skin could portend just about anything. It could be mild but annoying, such as the enterovirus (hand, foot, and mouth disease) or varicella zoster virus (chicken pox), or it could be lethal and potentially highly transmissible, such as the herpesvirus B (encephalomyelitis) or the variola virus (smallpox).

He chimes in, "I had treated a herpes B-infected human while in New York."

According to Dr Yeo, macaque species were assumed to be positive for herpesvirus B unless proven otherwise. This, however, was not the case for orangutans. For them, the veterinarians were mostly concerned with diseases such as tuberculosis that were transmitted via the respiratory route. In fact, as veterinarians, their utmost concern was for reverse zoonosis or zooanthroponosis — human visitors infecting the apes. Several of the apes would often come down with the cold after crowded events, such as photography sessions with the orangutans. As a fascinating insight, the upper eyelids of the apes are used to perform skin tests for tuberculosis, unlike humans, where the test is performed on their forearms. It was a matter of hirsutism.

Back to David, who had chuckled at our impressive differentials of vesicular lesions. "I didn't identify intracellular inclusions or anything unusual on the Tzanck prep. The baby also had oral ulcers. Her signs and symptoms resolved within a few days without intervention. I suspect she possibly had an enterovirus or Herpesviridae. And the mother didn't kill me, which was fortunate, because they're very protective. The guards were saying, '*Look, doctor, watch out, because she will crush your head.*' So anyway, that part worked out okay." We knew that veterinarians were at risk of being bitten or scratched by their patients, but being pulverised? That was a different equation altogether.

Dr Yeo immediately pointed out to us that, except for the full-grown adult males, the other orangutans, adult females, sub-adults and infants, were handled by keepers. They were thus able to examine the infant without having to separate it from the mother, nor was any sedation necessary for the mother. This would not be the case for most, if not all, US zoos, where staff do not share the same space with apes without some form of anaesthesia. It was an occupational hazard.

David pressed on with his next consult. "The next one I saw was a teenage orangutan male who had bacterial meningitis. I managed to successfully perform an LP on him. It was not straightforward to do. The usual landmark, which is the iliac crest, goes up to the scapula in orangutans. So you couldn't really use that." In humans, the needle is inserted at the lumbar region, hence the name lumbar puncture, with the iliac crest being used as a landmark. Inserting it between the shoulder blades would risk causing lower limb paralysis. "I had to get two keepers to bend the orangutan to access a path to the thecal sac. He had opisthotonus [severe backward arching from neck to heel] when I saw him. The guards were able to flex his spine which was quite a feat. I managed to LP him, and when I saw the fluid in the LP, I was relieved. We then started an intravenous drip in his ankle and gave him ceftriaxone [an antibiotic]." Dr Yeo recalled that the orangutan was so stiff, he was unable to lie flat on his back, and they ended up having to build a wooden platform to support him in a sitting position.

Prof Brenda Ang had been an unwitting 'accomplice' to this as well.[30] One incident that had always stuck on her mind was seeing David in the equipment room in Ward 48, SGH, looking for a lumbar puncture needle. This would have been an unusual sight — it was an anomaly for a medical consultant to hunt for medical equipment, let alone perform routine procedures that were typically handled by junior doctors. Asked to explain himself, he sheepishly revealed that he needed something long enough to do an LP on a gorilla in the Singapore Zoo. It eventually turned out to be an orangutan, though the procedure was correct.

David continued with the case discussion. "Never grew anything from the cerebrospinal fluid, unfortunately. I don't know why. I don't know if the time it took to get the specimens to the lab was the reason or not. I assumed it was pneumococcus. But he improved despite our difficulties keeping an intravenous catheter in him." It was a triumph.

For Dr Yeo, this was one of those rare instances where an animal had a successful recovery after a severe disease. Often, the issue was detected too late as wild animals hide their clinical signs as a defensive behaviour. They, his keepers and her, were close to tears the day he was well enough to finally stand up. Years later, when she returned for a visit, he was still alive, and if for a very imperceptible occasional tongue protrusion, one would not have known he ever had meningitis.

We moved on to David's third and final case. "The third one was a great ape — a gorilla. And he was in extremis when I arrived. He was a young male, I think in his teens. But he was in septic shock. He was one of the last great apes that we had, and he died of melioidosis. The blood cultures grew *Burkholderia pseudomallei* [the causative agent of melioidosis]. I gave him ceftazidime, but he was already gone. It was enormously sad." Dr Yeo added that the necropsy performed on the gorilla revealed numerous 5–10 mm granulomas throughout the lungs, which was a feature typical of melioidosis.

David then brought up an interesting fact. "Many of them, if not all of them, had melioidosis. And that's why we're discouraged from hosting great apes." The Singapore Zoo used to keep gorillas in captivity, but the majority of them eventually became infected with and succumbed to *B. pseudomallei*, which is commonly found in the soil. Four gorillas in 1984, and another in 1992, died from the disease. The remaining one, imported in 1992, was quickly returned to the Dublin Zoo the year after its arrival.[38] Dr Yeo shared with us that all manner of precautions had been taken at the zoo, such as disinfecting the leafy branches, also known as browse, before the gorillas had access to them, in addition to housing them in an exhibit with concrete flooring and not natural substrate, since the pathogen was ubiquitous in the soil and water. However, it ultimately proved to be futile.

David was happy to call time on his veterinarian adventures following that, and for which Dr Yeo was grateful for all his assistance provided. "This was the dawn of Infectious Diseases in Singapore, but I'm sure now they have vets who are comfortable with the antibiotics available to them. I never treated a reptile, never treated a bird. Thank goodness." We were bemused — even he had limits on whom or what he would treat.

Four years pass and he's managed to accomplish his goal of setting up clinical Infectious Diseases services in Singapore, including the first department of Infectious Diseases at TTSH in 1992. Having barely got started, his oeuvre still in its infancy, he decides that he's had enough. Why did he leave this first-time round? Rumours have always abounded that it was because he felt disrespected, because he wasn't receiving the appropriate recognition and remuneration for what he brought to the table.

He parries the hearsay. "Honestly, I don't recall compensation as the issue. But, despite being faculty in the States, because of my age I was appointed as a senior resident in Singapore when I first arrived, which I wasn't terribly pleased about at the time. But I became a consultant after that, so that was okay. I just thought my initial appointment was based on age, not capacity. In every workplace we should focus less on a person's age, and more on what she or he can bring to the table. Anyway, so no, I don't recall compensation or a sense of being disrespected as being a factor." It would seem that there were some partial truths in the rumour.

He gives his side of the story on why he left. "My parents were getting older. I'm the third of three boys. The need to help my parents as they aged was on my mind." Reasons of family aside, the truth of his first departure was still down to a matter of exasperation, that he was constantly tackling a Sisyphean task. "I felt that I couldn't say no to anything. I felt my obligation was to say yes to everything, for fear of turning down something that would leave a bad taste in a decision maker's mind. So I took on more and more in Singapore. There were some lingering frustrations. *'We're providing services and doing more beyond our mandate. Help us to grow.'* And the response was, *'Bide your time.'* There were some professional frustrations there. As much as I say I understood it, and I did, it was still very frustrating, to be working hard, and feel that more time would be required before we're able to expand, whether it's Infection Prevention and Control, whether it's being allotted more trainees. It was frustrating."

"So that's why I left. I thought I saw an academic window in the US closing. The trajectory of getting things done when I first came to Singapore was very steep, and then it began to level off. I felt I was in an unstable situation in Singapore and so the question was, *'Do I continue to try to push things along here'* or have I lost my effectiveness and, *'Step away and let someone else try.'* I also saw the opportunity for resuming an academic career in the US closing if I waited too long. So that was that."

And so he handed over the reins of the ID department to Dr Wong Sin Yew, and then closed the door on Singapore. Only to find the auspices back home not particularly hospitable either.

"Little did I know that the window had closed already, in the US. I was naïve to think when I left New York for Singapore in 1989 that I'm going to show them, I'm going to come here [Singapore], I'm going to leave such a body of work, and programmes in place, that when I go back, my old institution is going to embrace me. I went back to the US for a variety of reasons. At the end of four years, I went back and they said, *'You can have your old job.'* I said, *'Well, I'm four years older. I've been a Head of a department, which I set up, I've trained people, we've published, we've effective programmes in place.'*"

And his past decision to leave comes back to haunt him.

"'But you did not do it under us. So, you've been dead to us for four years. You will be put back on the same committees you were on before you left, and you'll take your place on the tenure track where you were when you left.' Okay, so I went to see the Godfather, who'd moved on to industry then. And he said, *'You shouldn't have done it.'* I said, *'Really? I did all this!'* And he goes, *'It's not the way it's done.'*"

It was a bitter blow. "I decided not to return to New York Hospital. I took a year off and backpacked through Indonesia."

Following that, he had multiple job offers, but ended up in Texas, where his old medical school had been. "Here was a guy, Steven Seidenfeld, a New Yorker, ID-trained and living in Texas, who'd gone into private practice. He is a unique character — smart, ethical, passionate, and urbane. He was based in a hospital where a bone marrow transplant program was expanding. Prior to joining, I met the bone marrow transplanter, Craig Rosenfeld, and expand the bone marrow transplant program, they did. I joined Dr Seidenfeld and eventually became the president and managing partner of that practice, and expanded it to seven ID physicians. We ended up providing ID consultation and management for 80 inpatient transplant beds, a very active outpatient stem cell transplant programme along with solid organ transplant recipients, and a busy general Infectious Diseases inpatient practice."

But it seems that the old adage of '*you can take the man out of Singapore, but you can never take Singapore out of the man*' held true for him.

"After being back in the States, I started coming back to Singapore intermittently, almost immediately. There were a couple of items with the Singapore Medical Council wanting ID expert opinion input. And then I'd come back to various Western Pacific meetings, or the equivalent of the Asia Pacific meetings. But those visits were sporadic until 2011. And then the Courage Fund invited me to visit for a few months a year. I started doing that, and realised that I wanted to spend even more time in Singapore."

Prof Paul Tambyah claims credit for formally bringing David back into the Singapore fold in 2011, after his long hiatus. It was a 'return' for the favour that David had done for him all those years back, having been a referee for his application for ID training in Chicago. Bedside clinical teaching in Singapore had been identified by successive generations of ID trainees as a gap, and he felt that David would be the person to fill that chasm. The Courage Fund Visiting Professorship/Fellowship in Infectious Disease and Epidemiology (2004) was set up specifically to enable NUS to appoint eminent international experts in the field of ID to share their experiences and expertise here in Singapore.[39]

David similarly concurs. "Paul Ananth shared that he felt I provided perspectives and a teaching style which would benefit Singapore trainees as well as post-specialist training ID faculty. It was discussed for some time [before he agreed to coming back]. I needed to assure my time in Singapore did not compromise my ability to fulfil obligations in the US." Beyond that, and similar to his first outing, he had no qualms about packing his bags and leaving his career in US behind to come back to this sunny island. "It came at a good point in my professional life. I had achieved what I wanted to achieve professionally in Dallas and I did not feel sad stepping away from leading the group. I had extensive experience handling complex cases — strategies, coordinating professional alliances, defining success. My thoughts were that sharing the lessons learned would be beneficial to Singapore ID physicians to accelerate their evolution."

In 2016, Prof Hsu Li Yang, who was then the Head of Infectious Diseases at TTSH/CDC, further negotiated a deal for him to come to Singapore for up to 6-9 months each year so that the younger generation of ID physicians and trainees could have a more 'sustained exposure' to him.[40] The Courage Fund trips prior to that had only been for short periods of 2-3 months each. Prof Hsu believed that David would bring about stronger collegial mentorship and be a clinical exemplar, which was important for a clinical ID community that was growing more fragmented. David didn't bat an eyelid. "The message, since 2011, has always been that I'm here to be of service, and to provide one example of a long, varied and fulfilling career in Infectious Diseases."

Were there any 'stern' warnings, in a similar vein to his first stint, from the partners in his practice?

"They did not believe I was serious until I insisted that they transition into executive positions in the practice, and I referred decision making regarding administrative issues to them. They were not as excited about my time in Singapore as I was."

Coming back to the topic — why did he *want* to come back, though?

"The problem is teaching. I gave it up, and I realised how much I missed it. I wasn't doing that in private practice." He had missed teaching. "I had approached the medical school from which I had graduated to offer myself as a teacher. I had a transactional relationship with the Head of ID at that time, prior to Trish Perl's tenure, not a personal one — she was interested, but the atmosphere was not one of mutual respect. The ID Division of University of Texas Southwestern Graduate Medical School was not able to provide a comparable opportunity."

He was well aware of what was wanted of him. "Singapore was not interested in me as a researcher or administrator or a clinician, necessarily. Teaching was what was being sought from me." We'd missed his teaching as well. "It's the way *you* [referring to Gabriel] teach, which is engaging, making it a dynamic process." Here, we quote Prof Brenda Ang about what exactly David brings to the table — '*Most importantly…he's made it fun and enjoyable to see cases with him.*[30]'

And so that's how we've all ended up here, in this room, having this conversation. His visceral need to educate the next generation of Infectious Diseases specialists, and more, in Singapore.

Looking back, were there any regrets about his original endeavour, back in 1989? Did he have any advice to give to his younger self, and therefore, in some ways, to us?

"Don't agree to do everything that's asked of you, to seek endorsement and approval. You don't have to do that. That's what I did not understand as a young person. I thought I had to say yes to everything in an effort to legitimize my bigger goals. It was painful. It certainly helped the process, but it also was exhausting and certainly shortened the period of time that I was here, sadly. When I would have rather stayed."

There's a lot to take in from this statement. In a bid to find relevance, and in part because of his personality, David was never disinclined to offer his talents when sought. But in doing so, he had spread himself too thin and, dare we say, potentially been exploited. It is a bit of an irony too that he could insouciantly brush away the intimidations of authority, but easily succumb to the charms of *cris de cœur*. Even now, we're not entirely sure if David would ever say no to anyone when his help was sought — we didn't think he could help himself. But it is precisely because of this that we are now the beneficiaries of his tireless efforts. As Friedrich Nietzsche, the German philosopher, once said, '*He who has a why to live can bear almost any how.*' That's how David lives.

We take another breather here and move on to something more light-hearted. By now, David would have lived in Singapore, accumulatively, for more than a decade and a half. We decided to quiz him on how naturalized he had become.

First off, when he spoke Singlish, was he trying to be funny, or was it second nature to him?

"It is reasonably natural to me. My friends will tell me just don't bother. The children of my friends just tell me to give it up. But no, it comes naturally to me."

His Singlish does come across as a little jarring. He's honed it over the years, one can tell. The tone is correct, the pronunciation is pristine, and the grammar is proper. But what gives it away is that it is admixed within an American-accented speech. And it doesn't help that he only has an almighty grin on his face every time he throws one in with comedic timing. Full marks for the effort though.

How about durians — does it taste like sweet custard ice-cream, or does it smell like a gas leak?

"I enjoy durian, but I will tell you, I will not go out and buy it. Because I'm afraid, if I buy it, I'll bring it to someone's house, or they'll come over and eat the durian, and invariably they will say, '*Oh, you've got the wrong durian*.'"

We clarified that it's like wine though — he just needs to go for the most expensive one.

"It's this durian snobbery that is just uncalled for. So sometimes I just don't bother."

This definitely won't sit well with the authorities, whoever they were. We move on to the next question.

Singaporeans like to queue for the sake of queuing — if he saw a long queue without knowing what's at the front, would he join it, or ignore it?

"Depends on how much time I have. I'm a bit more discerning, but yes, I'm aware that obviously someone's on to something. And I will look." He cites a recent example for us. "The other day, I took my brother and sister-in-law, who were in town, to Maxwell Food Centre, because we happened to be in the area. There was the chicken rice place there, but the queue was long. So, we bought chicken rice at one of the other stalls. And you know, my guests don't know any better. My brother said it was good."

We glowered. That was not okay at all. Guests in our country should only consume the finest hawker food, and the length of the queue correlated directly with its quality.

Did he at least *chope*[41] the table with a packet of tissue paper?

"With that day, I did it with my sunglasses and my hat. So, I definitely *chope*. I am *kiasu*,[42] no doubt. Actually, I was someplace yesterday with my brother and sister-in-law and I was about to *chope* with my wallet, but I thought, no, not even in Singapore would I do that. I'm sure nobody would take it, but it's a little risky."

He's redeemed himself a little with that. What else did he appreciate about Singaporean culture?

"I like the notion where a good evening is going to somebody's house, or have somebody come to your place. You sit around in your shorts. You tell stories. You have some food. You play mahjong." Bonus points for that. "You sit around with your buddies and you chit chat. And you just enjoy each other's company. That part of Singapore culture I really like."

He passes the test, but only just. All jokes aside, we were glad that he was one of us.

Before we moved on to the next topic, we had one last curiosity to satisfy. We return back to his role as an educator. What was his *modus operandi* in training someone to become an ID physician? How does one fashion a slab of marble into a masterpiece?

"By standing shoulder to shoulder with each generation. We [him and the trainees] are made the same, and our goals are similar. I've travelled similar paths to what they are travelling. The secret sauce is transforming those experiences into practical lessons — patient care, professional development, and our duties as ID physicians."

He was paternal in nature, but not in approach. Pedagogic but not didactic. Us succeeding would mean that he had similarly succeeded. And for that, he wanted his experiences to be ours as well.

Notes

[1] There are four types of influenza viruses — A, B, C, and D. Pandemics are typically caused by the influenza A virus, and seasonal flu by influenza A and B viruses. Influenza C viruses generally cause mild illness, and influenza D viruses typically affect only cattle with no known transmission to humans. Influenza A viruses are further subtyped according to two proteins found on their surface — haemagglutinin (H) and neuraminidase (N), of which there are 18 and 11 different subtypes for the former and the latter respectively.

[2] K. S. Loh and L. Y. Hsu. (2023) Pandemics in Singapore, 1819–2022 (Routledge Studies in the Modern History of Asia). Routledge.

[3] M. Honigsbaum. 'Revisiting the 1957 and 1968 influenza pandemics', *Lancet*. 2020 Jun 13;395(10240):1824–1826.

[4] Polio and The Epidemic Intelligence Service (EIS). CDC. [https://www.cdc.gov/museum/online/story-of-cdc/polio/index.html] (accessed 31 Jan 2024)

[5] L. H. Lee and K. A. Lim. 'Eradication of poliomyelitis in Singapore', *Singapore Med J*. 1977 Mar;18(1):34–40.

[6] M. A. Riva. 'From milk to rifampicin and back again: history of failures and successes in the treatment for tuberculosis', *J Antibiot (Tokyo)*. 2014 Sep;67(9):661–5.

[7] MRCI. 'Streptomycin Treatment of Pulmonary Tuberculosis', *Br Med J*. 1948 Oct 30;2(4582):769–82.

[8] STS/BH/BMRCI. 'A controlled clinical trial of the role of thiacetazone-containing regimens in the treatment of pulmonary tuberculosis in Singapore', *Tubercle*. 1971 Jun;52(2):88–116.

[9] STS/BMRC 'Controlled trial of intermittent regimens of rifampicin plus isoniazid for pulmonary tuberculosis in Singapore', *Lancet*. 1975 Dec 6;2(7945):1105–9.

[10] STS/BMRC 'Clinical trial of six-month and four-month regimens of chemotherapy in the treatment of pulmonary tuberculosis', *Am Rev Respir Dis*. 1979 Apr;119(4):579–85.

[11] W. Fox et al. 'Studies on the treatment of tuberculosis undertaken by the British Medical Research Council tuberculosis units, 1946–1986, with relevant subsequent publications', *Int J Tuberc Lung Dis*. 1999 Oct; 3(10 Suppl 2):S231–79.

12 HDB begins selling flats under home ownership scheme. NLB. [https://www.nlb.gov.sg/main/article-detail?cmsuuid=2ab696d3-d9f5-4970-9108-e0f95919cc98#3] (accessed 31 Jan 2024)

13 K. S. Loh and L. Y. Hsu. (2019) Tuberculosis — the Singapore Experience, 1867–2018: Disease, Society and the State (Routledge Studies in the Modern History of Asia). Routledge.

14 The History and Evolution of Singapore's Hawker Culture. Roots. [https://www.roots.gov.sg/stories-landing/stories/Serving-Up-a-Legacy] (accessed 31 Jan 2024)

15 Typhoid. NLB. [https://www.nlb.gov.sg/main/article-detail?cmsuuid=d84fdf0f-34a2-4cc0-8930-47d2ff9dacd0] (accessed 31 Jan 2024)

16 Journeys of Transformation: Singapore's Pig Farmers after Pig Farming. SFA. 8 Sep 2022. [https://www.sfa.gov.sg/food-for-thought/article/detail/journeys-of-transformation-singapore's-pig-farmers-after-pig-farming]

17 Of Swine and Sustainability Change, Choices, and Challenges of Pig Farming in Singapore, 1965–1984, Roots. [https://www.roots.gov.sg/stories-landing/stories/of-swine-and-sustainability/story] (accessed 31 Jan 2024)

18 Y. L. Koh et al. 'Japanese encephalitis, Singapore', *Emerg Infect Dis*. 2006 Mar;12(3):525–6.

19 E. See et al. 'Presence of hemagglutination inhibition and neutralization antibodies to Japanese encephalitis virus in wild pigs on an offshore island in Singapore', *Acta Trop*. 2002 Mar;81(3):233–6. doi: 10.1016/s0001-706x(01)00212-1.

20 S. H. L. Ting et al. 'Seroepidemiology of neutralizing antibodies to Japanese encephalitis virus in Singapore: continued transmission despite abolishment of pig farming?', *Acta Trop*. 2004 Nov–Dec;92(3):187–91.

21 V. G. Heiser. (1936) An American Doctor's Odyssey: Adventures in Forty-Five Countries. W W Norton & Co Inc.

22 Interview with Prof John Wong [14 Feb 2024]

23 Email interview with Prof Chee Yam Cheng [20 Nov 2023]

24 Human Manpower Development Programme. Launched in the 1980s by MOH, it was a scheme to provide local specialists the opportunity to train and work at renowned healthcare institutes worldwide.

25 Tan Tock Seng Hospital

26 Singapore General Hospital

27 Which APAC countries are the most overworked in 2022? Instant Offices. 6 Jun 2022. [https://www.instantoffices.com/blog/featured/most-overworked-apac-countries/] (accessed 31 Jan 2024)

28 Anti-yellow culture campaign. NLB. [https://www.nlb.gov.sg/main/article-detail?cmsuuid=8e493ee4-1832-4fec-96ee-a0a6b3efab87] (accessed 29 Feb 2024)

29 Email interview with Prof Raymond Lin [23 Nov 2023]

30 Email interview with Prof Brenda Ang [9 Dec 2023]

31 Society of Infectious Disease (Singapore)

32 The Silence that Preceded China's Great Leap into Famine. Smithsonian Magazine. 26 Sep 2012. [https://www.smithsonianmag.com/history/the-silence-that-preceded-chinas-great-leap-into-famine-51898077/]

33 Recommendations from My Bookshelf: Cutting for Stone by Abraham Verghese. ASH Clinical News. [https://ashpublications.org/ashclinicalnews/news/2506/Recommendations-from-My-Bookshelf-Cutting-for] (accessed 31 Jan 2024)

34 Email interview with Prof Chong Chia Yin [19 Feb 2024]

35 An Indonesian hideaway fit for a princess? SCMP. 22 Aug 1993. [https://www.scmp.com/article/41265/indonesian-hideaway-fit-princess#amp_tf=From%20%251%24s&aoh=17065966865475&referrer=https%3A%2F%2Fwww.google.com&share=https%3A%2F%2Fwww.scmp.com%2Farticle%2F41265%2Findonesian-hideaway-fit-princess]

36 How Dinosaurs Shrank and Became Birds. Scientific American. 12 Jun 2015. [https://www.scientificamerican.com/article/how-dinosaurs-shrank-and-became-birds/]

37 Email interview with Dr Shirey Yeo [04 Mar 2024]

38 S. H. Sim et al. 'Melioidosis in Singapore: Clinical, Veterinary, and Environmental Perspectives', *Trop Med Infect Dis.* 2018 Mar 12;3(1):31.

39 Professorships. NUS. [https://nus.edu.sg/nusgiving/named-professorships] (accessed 31 Jan 2024)

40 Email interview with Prof Hsu Li Yang [20 Nov 2023]

41 Hokkien term for reserving a seat.

42 Hokkien term for being afraid to lose out.

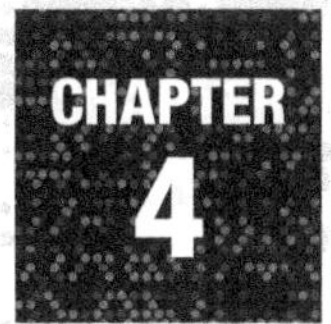

PLAGUES

—

saepe ne utile quidem est scire quid futurum sit
'often, it is not advantageous to know what will be'

The English word 'plague' is derived from the Latin word *'plaga'*, which means *'blow'* or *'wound'*. To Biblical scholars, the word 'plague' is synonymous with Moses and the book of Exodus in the Torah. The wrath of God was inflicted upon the Egyptians who had kept His people, the Jews, under the tyranny of slavery. This decade of plagues included turning the waters of the river Nile into blood, indiscriminately unleashing frogs, lice, flies, livestock pestilence, boils, hail, locusts, and darkness upon the land, and finally, the killing of every firstborn son not protected by the hand of God. 'Plague' in this context, translated from the Hebrew word 'נגף' [*negef*], means *'to strike down'* — in this sense, it was a supernatural affliction exacted upon its victims. It did not connote any particular human disease.

To a Shakespearean bardolator, the 'plague' is the defining prophecy in *'Romeo and Juliet'*. Mercutio, Romeo's best friend, unleashes the infamous curse, *'a plague o' both your houses'*, after being mortally wounded by Juliet's cousin, Tybalt, whilst defending Romeo's honour. The multi-generational feud between the Montagues and the Capulets resulted in the futile loss of his life, and in this instance, the 'plague' is a curse of calamity, foretelling the tragic demise of the play's protagonists. Curiously, the word 'pox', alluding to smallpox, is used interchangeably with the word 'plague' in different versions of the play, implying that the Bard himself ascribed no particular contagion to this curse.[1]

Used in an English idiomatic expression such as '*to avoid like the plague*', the 'plague' here refers to '*a disastrous evil or affliction*' or '*a cause of irritation*' which is to be steered clear of. As for the Dutch, whose language of insults and expletives is intimately tied to diseases, the 'plague' is used in a couple of ways. A '*pestkop*', or a '*plague head*', is a derisive term for a '*bully*'. '*De pest in hebben*', or '*to have the plague in*', is a slang for being '*in a bad mood*'. To the Russians, a 'plague' would mean a minor irritation. 'Просто чума' [*prosto chuma*], or Russian for '*just a plague*', is a colloquial expression meaning '*it was crazy*' or '*holy-moly*', and is generally used to make light of a bad situation. In Chinese, the old idiom '义不容辞' [yì bù róng cí], which describes the feeling of something being mandatory, received a new update following the COVID-19 pandemic. The first character, '义', which means '*obligation*', is replaced with a similar sounding word '疫', meaning 'plague'. '疫不容辞' [yì bù róng cí] hence describes the determination of the medical staff, and the nation as a whole, striving against a new invisible threat.

For an Infectious Diseases specialist, there is but one true 'plague' — the disease caused by the bacterium *Yersinia pestis*. It is synonymous with the 'Black Death', a 14th century, catastrophic event in human history where up to a third of the population in Europe perished. It is most recognisable by the blood-curdling beak-shaped face mask adorned by plague doctors, with its snout filled with aromatic herbs and medicament which purportedly sterilised the inhaled miasma, creating a protective aura around its wearer. Three forms of plagues exist — bubonic plague, the most common presentation, is characterised by swollen, painful lymph nodes called buboes; septicaemic plague, occurring when the bacteria multiply within the bloodstream; and the pneumonic plague, the deadliest version, for which a rapidly progressive and fatal pneumonia is a prominent feature. The bubonic and septicaemic plagues typically develop following the bite of infected rodent fleas, whilst the pneumonic plague is transmitted from person-to-person through the inhalation of infected respiratory secretions. It was this latter form that ravaged the Chinese population in the Manchurian Black Death of 1910, killing more than 60,000 people in the north-eastern Chinese province. The outbreak was only halted following the institution of various public health measures, including mask wearing and isolation protocols, by a Penang-born Chinese doctor, Dr Wu Lien-Teh. He astutely recognised this outbreak to encompass only the pneumonic and not the bubonic form of the plague, and recommended that the authorities and general public abandon the futile hunt for rats harbouring fleas. Instead, he advocated the use of a self-constructed rudimentary gauze-and-cotton mask which has now evolved to become the medical masks that we now commonly wear to prevent the transmission of airborne diseases. He may not have invented the face mask, but he was a pioneer in its use for the effective prevention of contagion.

In Jonathan Kennedy's historically sweeping book '*Pathogenesis*', which views human history through microbial lenses, he contends that *Homo sapiens* 'very often…don't make history in circumstances of our own choosing, but in circumstances created by microbes'.[2] Infectious diseases have very often been the king makers in the history of humanity. In Neolithic times, zoonotic diseases, in particular the plague, were harboured by early farmers, herders and their livestock from Anatolia and the Great Steppe, and carried into Europe. This decimated the indigenous European hunter-gatherers, leading to the rise of sedentary agricultural societies. Sustained attacks by the plague also weakened the stranglehold of the Roman empire, allowing the Ottoman empire to become the dominant hegemony of the Old World. Across the Atlantic, it was smallpox that led the charge for the Spanish conquistadors, and together with other infectious diseases such as measles and influenza, obliterated the indigenous population of Mesoamerica in the 16th century, whose population declined from a peak of 20 million to 1.5 million within a century. The dynasties of the New World were thus laid low by Old World pathogens. Infectious diseases have plagued mankind since its existence, and will never cease to shape the course of human history. Which leads us to our topic for this section of the discourse — we probed David's thoughts on the most recent plague of the Anthropocene age, COVID-19, and further explore what future plagues humankind may be beset with, and how best we can lay the groundwork for them now.

We are now in 2023 and the trajectory which the COVID-19 pandemic took, and will take, has become clearer with the passage of time. The history of COVID-19 is relatively well known to all, so recent is this plague of our times, but it is still worth recounting for posterity. What started out as a cluster of unknown respiratory illnesses stemming from a wet market in Wuhan, China, in late December 2019, quickly engulfed the rest of the world in 2020, and brought its many vibrant economies to its knees. Caused by the virus SARS-CoV-2,[3] a relative of the original SARS[4] and MERS[5] coronaviruses, it was highly transmissible and sufficiently virulent enough to overwhelm hospitals with the sick and the dying. As such, to protect these indispensable national pillars, governments all over the world were compelled to erect barriers preventing personnel entering the country from abroad, and imposing lockdowns on its own population so as to 'flatten the curve'.[6] In the dealings with such a novel pathogen, no treatments or vaccinations were initially available, and age-old measures such as quarantine, epidemiological surveillance, and isolation,[7] together with masking and social distancing, were utilised as blunt tools to combat this pandemic. It was only with the arrival of effective vaccines, at the end of 2020, did it spell the beginning of the pandemic's end. By the end of December 2023, there have been at least 7 million deaths from COVID-19, out of a total of 773 million confirmed cases worldwide.[8] The COVID-19 pandemic has now moved on to its next phase, with the population learning to live with its endemicity. The number of infections continue to wax and wane with each new variant surfacing and the population learning to adapt to it, either through natural infections or with vaccination boosters. Indeed, the turbulent times at the beginning of the pandemic seem like distant memories to us now, but we revisit the moment again, wondering how David viewed this whole sequence of events with the sagacity accumulated over his years operating out in the field.

How did he first get wind of the news and what were the immediate thoughts that crossed his mind?

"I was in Dallas. I read it on ProMED Mail.org and thought, '*Hmmm, this information sounds suspicious*.'" ProMED, which is short for 'Program for Monitoring Emerging Diseases', is the largest publicly-available surveillance system conducting global reporting of infectious diseases outbreaks. "Larry Madoff was one of my medical residents at New York Hospital when I was an intern. As Editor of ProMed Mail.org, Larry wrote interesting commentaries, so I read ProMED mail religiously as a lurker."

Was he afraid that things were going to get bad very quickly?

"I thought it would become clear quickly whether the report was '*noise*' or '*signal*'. The events did not evoke fear. I was scheduled to begin my next Courage Fund posting in Singapore on 27th January 2020. I received a message from John Eu Li Wong in mid-January, before the first case in Singapore, letting me know that if I wanted to cancel my trip to Singapore because of the potential risks, I could." He didn't. By then, this mysterious illness was known to be caused by a novel coronavirus, and based on historical evidence provided by the original SARS, it had the potential to wrought a lot of havoc. Wasn't he concerned about his own safety? "I was not. Being aware of what one doesn't know is almost as empowering as knowing."

Like many of us, he would not have been able to know that it would be more than two years later before the storm had passed, before he was able to step foot out of this sunny island again. Before we ventured in depth about the plague of our times, we queried first his experiences dealing with pandemics or outbreaks in the past.

"I've found the work and detail required to prepare and respond to outbreaks professionally satisfying. These included, more recently in Dallas, influenza in 2009 and Ebola in 2014. They require your full attention and were important diversions from the day-to-day routine of an ID physician." He was not the least bit dismayed at having to face yet another potential disaster. Instead, it connected right to his core — he found relevance. "They give the ID community an opportunity to display the broader spectrum of their skills and their value to the ecosystem."

Since no two pandemics are truly alike, how did his past experiences in dealing with one help with the COVID-19 pandemic?

"Be calm. Don't act before you have sufficient factual information. Also, you'll never have all you want. Prioritise what needs to be done, communicate clearly, be confident in the process and at the same time express humility that well-intentioned mistakes will be made and corrected."

We decided to play the devil's advocate. During the initial stages of the COVID-19 pandemic, when the virus was still a relatively unknown entity, the government and the medical community were wading through a fog. The old playbook from the original SARS outbreak in 2002 was dusted off and utilised, but it ultimately proved ineffective in containing the spread. As an example, those infected with the original SARS virus were only contagious when they were symptomatic, and we initially based our COVID-19 contact tracing on this evidence. However, it was subsequently found that COVID-19 patients were actually contagious up to 48 hours prior to the onset of symptoms. As a result, we had been letting many through the quarantine net based on a false assumption. To be fair, we wouldn't have known any better till the necessary evidence had been gathered. Were past experiences in handling outbreaks actually of any utility, or more of a hindrance because it gave false reassurances?

"Useful. They are premised on our conceptual understanding at the time they are made, and biased toward zero collateral damage. We learn and modify as we go. If resources are nil or limited at the onset, we might reset the calculus regarding what constitutes acceptable collateral damage."

The picture painted seemed a little too rosy. Even during the outbreak of Zika in Singapore in 2018, we had been isolating infected patients in healthcare facilities until they tested negative. At least initially. These policies were, seemingly to us, haphazardly adopted from SARS, which spread from person-to-person via respiratory particles, onto a virus which spread mostly with the aid of a vector, the mosquito. As an aside, other ways by which the Zika virus could be transmitted between persons was through sexual contact, and from a mother to her child *in utero*.

"Policy is a product of science and politics. We, as healthcare providers are science-based people and generally don't have dual roles as politicians. Politics will take care of itself. That is why we have people who are professionals at politics. They can be advised from the science available, and understand what their [the scientist's] perceptions are, what the instruments of government available are, and then try to wed those, and realise that policy which results will not be perfect. But it is okay, we can change it as more information becomes available. I do not underestimate the difficulty policymakers face."

But the fact of the matter was that adopting policies from a previous pandemic didn't seem to work, and so, what was its true value?

"But do you think it didn't work for lack of effort? There definitely was effort, but it was a flawed model. How many times had we experienced COVID-19? So, all we can do is to adjust on the fly. After the pandemic is less burdensome, we can review our successes and shortcomings, and learn from others experiences. How can we be more strategic in where we focus our investments, appreciating that our resources are finite? What can we do to mitigate harm to critical infrastructure and to people? While we can be intentional in future epidemic/pandemic preparedness, avoidance appears to be more a pipe-dream at this point in time, with early detection and limiting fallout the more realistic outcomes."

Another controversy that erupted during the pandemic had been that of mask-wearing. The initial stance from the authorities and experts was that there was little utility for wearing one, and some of those in the community who advocated for its use were publicly ridiculed.[9] Furthermore, masks had been quickly becoming short in supply, and the intention at the time had been to reserve this finite resource for where the need had been the greatest — in healthcare settings. This turned out to be a major gaffe, and the messaging changed once the science showed that mask-wearing was protective, but not before some reputational damage had been done. What were his thoughts on healthcare professionals who might otherwise vehemently disagree with policy and want to speak out, all for the oath they had sworn, to protect the safety of the patient, and hence the public?

Surprisingly, or perhaps unsurprisingly, David gives a politically correct answer. "Public health policy strives to optimize health outcomes for the greatest number of residents. Governments, who are the source of policy, have tacit and/or explicit social compacts with their citizens, which informs how policy decision making is achieved, debated and shared." He sidesteps this thorny issue. "I was not involved in the discussions. As such, I did not know the status of the specific logistical variables which factored into the equation — mask stockpiles, mask supply chain, masks needed — nor the ability to divert human resources from other pressing matters to assure mask compliance. These issues and others not mentioned are important components of decision making. My thoughts are irrelevant in the absence of knowing the facts available to those who made the decisions." We wonder if he would have answered us differently if we had conducted this interview in his country of birth. After all, if not for the HIV/AIDS activists in the United States who fought for their rights, we would not have seen the significant progress made in that field. Even Dr Anthony Fauci would attest to that.[10] We weren't advocating for picketing here in Singapore, and not that it would be tolerated either, but was there some other way beyond just toeing the line? We had placed David in a quagmire. "Government has a responsibility to do what governments are supposed to do, as its citizens have an expectation of what government is to do. I don't know how to answer this because I am outsider. Although I have been immersed in the Singapore medical scene since the late 1980s, I would like to think I have some perspective, but I bring the viewpoint that I was raised with, so it is a little tricky for me to answer."

Since we were on the topic of governance, how would he grade Singapore's performance during the COVID-19 pandemic?

"It's all relative. I have the luxury of being very familiar with how things transpired in the US and in Singapore, and I chose to be in Singapore, not because I am a martyr. I believe Singapore is a highly functioning society, one that I am thrilled to participate in. From the medical side, I was in contact with my colleagues in the US, and they were pulling their hair out, frustrated. I don't deny that there were frustrating things that occurred in Singapore as well, but I don't think that it was to the same degree as in the US. As information becomes available, policy evolves. One of the big differences between Singapore and the US in terms of how COVID-19 was handled was the constant communication in Singapore. To be honest with you, while I did receive many emails and texts every day from the Singapore Ministry of Health, and I may not have agreed with all of them, the information provided rational explanations for why certain policies were being implemented. Communications in the US were not as unified, co-ordinated, rational, or as frequent. Everyone's motives were questioned in the US. I understood the motives of the Singapore leadership. My observations are that the elected leaders in Singapore are representing what they believe, to the best of their abilities, to be in the best interest of Singaporeans, full stop."

In Singapore, our then Prime Minister Lee Hsien Loong, very early on in the pandemic, instituted a 'circuit breaker',[11] and called for members of the public to wear masks and adhere to social distancing.[12] In the States, President Trump lamented at press conferences that there was too much testing for COVID-19,[13] and also recklessly suggested that injecting disinfectant, or somehow inserting ultraviolet light into the body, could kill the virus.[14] It was not an entirely fair comparison, but he was right — the motives of our leadership could not be questioned. But still, could we have done better?

"I think we are more than capable, in Singapore, of interpreting data independently of others. Historically, we have looked outside for direction. We should continue to look outside at how others are approaching the same problem, and their rationale, but we should not take their assessment as the final word. We may not have access to the data available that others do, and we don't have the luxury of as many people working on the problem as others may. We may have more capable people per capita, but we don't have as many, in total. The lesson we have learnt is that we need to be as nimble, efficient and self-reliant as possible. This may be in the form of end-to-end vaccine development from ideation to commercialisation, or drug development, or public health."

Early on during the pandemic, Singapore was at the forefront globally in the fight against COVID-19. Besides receiving praise for how we were tackling the pandemic with rigorous contact tracing and flawless public communications,[15] we were leaders in the field of diagnostics as well. One of the diagnostic kits distributed globally, the Fortitude Kit, was made in Singapore. It was co-developed by A*STAR's Experimental Drug Development Centre, Bioinformatics Institute, and the Department of Laboratory Medicine at Tan Tock Seng Hospital.[16] As global supply chains turned inwards, our national stocks of nasal swabs for COVID-19 mass testing dwindled, and we turned inwards as well to look for ways to circumvent this issue. A solution was found at our local university using 3D-printing and injection moulding. A little-known fact — David had a significant hand in its production as well.[17] He was advocating for more of this sort of local industry and innovation in preparation for the future.

He went on. "In every aspect we need to be self-reliant, confident, and trust our process. Our process is one such that we make the best decision that we can, an earnest, thoughtful decision, based on the information available today. And we need to revisit this decision again on another day when more information becomes available. It is sometimes difficult to communicate these decisions to our stakeholders as the message may change along the way, but that's okay. That's what we need to do in the future, more of it — gather data, analyse, make a risk benefit assessment, take action and review outcomes. The confidence and speed in which those steps were taken accelerated as the pandemic evolved in Singapore."

We get him to elaborate — what was one such incident that impacted us negatively?

"Restricting testing. Who was to be tested and where they could be tested were initially pragmatic — restricted by case definition and finite testing capacity. But as capacity ramped up, access did not ramp up as quickly. As such, there were delays in mobilizing the private sector. The testing needs were greater than the public sector alone could manage."

One definite area for improvement was care for those living at the fringes of our society. It was a major blind spot of ours during the pandemic. Our migrant worker dormitories accommodated thousands of people, and once COVID-19 entered the premises, it spread like an uncontrollable wildfire till it had burnt out. To contain the spread, the workers were asked to practice social distancing, but it was akin to swimming with their limbs tied together. It was logistically impossible, as they continued to be housed in crowded and unsanitary conditions.[18] We explored a related issue of injustice to the migrant workers and how they were treated compared to the locals. There was a time during the pandemic when everyone who had COVID-19 was isolated, and Singaporeans who 'complained' may have been able to decline being 'decanted' to external facilities; whilst migrant workers, who did not have much of a voice, were all 'decanted' to other less comfortable facilities. What was his take on that?

"I think that's the issue of policy, which again results from a combination of science and politics. I personally found it challenging that people who did not need to be in the hospital, for a period of time, were able to say, *'I'm not leaving.'* Policy eventually caught up with the problem and provided us the support to expeditiously discharge them when they did not have a medical indication to be in hospital, even when they demanded to stay. But for a while, there were citizens and PR[19] and whomever, who stayed in hospital and denied that hospital bed to somebody in the ED[20] who needed it more than they did. And that was frustrating to me as a physician. So, I hear you, but policy caught up eventually. No system is perfect. I certainly think that my view should be the one that holds the day, but I understand that I work in a bigger healthcare system, and large organisations are generally not designed for immediacy of action. I'm not an apologist. I'm just trying to give perspective, because we in the trenches don't always see the whole priority picture."

We delve closer to home into more personal aspects of the pandemic, and how it affected the medical community. One such instance saw some medical departments ring-fence around their senior doctors and excused them from seeing patients who were suspected or confirmed to have COVID-19. A seemingly overabundance of precaution was taken to protect them, and this would have had a direct impact on David. Did he have an axe to grind, since he would have loved nothing better than to roll up his sleeves?

"I was not asked to participate in discussions or policy regarding COVID-19 patient care by senior clinicians. However, some of the thinking was shared with me. It was understandable to implement such a policy early in the pandemic as older persons were clearly at greater risk. But the position became less defensible as proven protection, vaccination and treatment evolved." We challenged further — should this then have been a decision left up to the individual? Though on the flip side, some of the more senior doctors may, in truth, want to avoid being put at risk, but also not appear as if they are not pulling their weight. If the department made that decision as a whole, this may then have lessened the guilt. "The individual is part of the department. I respect the department's sense of duty and responsibility. That said, it would have been nice to have the opportunity to participate in the discussion. I was able to directly and indirectly care for COVID-19 patients via NUH ID Department's rounding support provided to non-ID faculty-led primary COVID teams, 'COVID call' [providing over-the-phone consults on COVID-19 related matters], and my nasopharyngeal swab clinical trials. By the Delta wave, the hesitance to routinely involve senior clinicians had vanished." David rarely displays his grievances, but his reply bristled. This issue had clearly ruffled his feathers — he undoubtedly wanted in on more of the action, and had been limited from doing so early on.

During the original SARS outbreak, many healthcare professionals were pressured by their family members not to go to work, or to abstain from seeing infected patients, for fear of catching contagion. And even before that, when HIV first came onto the scenes in Singapore in the late 1980s, some doctors and nurses even actively discriminated against such patients by resigning or asking to be transferred elsewhere.[21] How does one strike a balance between the call of duty to patients, and the responsibilities to family, especially when one's life is at risk?

"That balance is a personal one, and is influenced by the opinion the physician has of their job. Is being a physician a calling, or the best option amongst many to occupy your time and provide for yourself and your family? A physician's work-life balance may change at different stages of his or her career. The traditional oaths taken by physicians upon graduation do not address selflessness, self-sacrifice or altruism in my reading." Healthcare professionals are humans after all, no matter how much we have been placed on a pedestal by the general public. Each individual has his or her own guiding principles, and they should not be faulted for following them.

A corollary of the COVID-19 pandemic was that it dulled the senses of the physicians without actually infecting them. One such manner was that, at the height of the pandemic, doctors were so inundated with COVID-19 patients that any patient who had a fever and was a possible contact, which was just about everyone, was immediately presumed to have COVID-19. Very occasionally it turned out not to be, with suspicions raised when the patient was not progressing like a typical case. Only then would an alternative diagnosis be sought, with a significant delay of a few days, which could potentially be detrimental to the patient.

"I agree with you. It has dulled the senses. Just like *Legionella* did, HIV, SARS, West Nile and MERS when they dominated Infectious Diseases physicians' worlds." These were the outbreaks of infectious diseases that occur once every couple of years — *Legionella* in the US in 1976, HIV beginning in 1981, West Nile in 1999, SARS in 2002, and MERS in 2012. Just to name a couple of them. "I think, certainly, because it is a common or has been a common diagnosis, it is foremost in people's mind. It is intruding on our thoughts, but I think it's only as much as you allow it to intrude. I try to listen to a story from a patient, or from a trainee, and I'm listening for a syndromic history and physical findings that will point our team in the correct direction, not a pre-determined direction."

He adds to the point. "But I think it has changed, in the sense, that there are several years of Infectious Diseases trainees whose training have been heavily coloured by having COVID-19 around..." He pauses here to shed light on his own experiences. "As my training was coloured by having the discovery and the management of a large number of HIV patients in the days before treatment. So I was heavily influenced by that. I think COVID-19 has changed what we do. But the day-to-day practice, it's still — take a history, do a physical examination, obtain the appropriate laboratory tests, synthesize appropriate differential diagnoses, and off you go." What he was emphasizing was the need to get our fundamentals right.

The management of COVID-19 patients also became algorithmic, and necessarily so. As we learnt more about the virus over time, we had to adapt our protocols to containing it. Patients were placed into high- or low-risk categories based on certain characteristics such as age and comorbidities. Treatment would only be initiated for patients who fulfilled a certain severity scoring criterion, and different forms of treatment were instituted dependent on the day of their infection and their oxygen requirements. It got even more convoluted once vaccinations came about. There was further risk stratification for instituting treatment, based on the type and number of vaccinations a person had. And all that was just treatment alone. Discharging patients was another ordeal of mental sums, governed by the day of illness, health and vaccination status of the patient, site of discharge (such as going home or to a community facility), and a crude estimate of the viral load. If people in the community found the rules for the public difficult to follow, it was even more bewildering for the healthcare worker.

Algorithmic management of our patients was complex, but then again, it was also unexacting because it took away any intuition a physician may have, and limited the thought processes he or she needed to make. What was David's perspective on this?

"Algorithms have been shown to overall improve quality of care. I'm not talking about just infectious diseases, but flying airplanes and performing surgery, and many other clinical activities." This was the premise of the book, '*The Checklist Manifesto*', by Atul Gawande. "But what I think is that we've allowed algorithms to inappropriately make us comfortable turning off our brains. Algorithms are meant to bring the least of us up to a competency level, but we can't allow algorithms to make the best of us mediocre. Algorithms depend on a certain basic science, an understanding of disease and agreed upon treatment strategies contemporary to the time the algorithm was developed. It's our job as thinking physicians to extrapolate what algorithms and guidelines tell us and say, '*It is appropriate for my patient to follow this algorithm to the letter, or it would be contrary to my patient's best interest to follow this algorithm because of my patient's unique features.*' So, I think algorithms are great for exams and for giving us a functional competence, but I think they have the potential, if one allows them to, to neuter excellence. I don't think this is unique to COVID-19. Algorithms exist and are used in managing *Staphylococcus aureus* bacteraemia, and in managing most if not all conditions we confront. I'm not saying algorithms are bad. I'm just saying that the algorithms need to be thoughtfully applied or varied from according to the patient's circumstances."

At the core of it all is an inherent fear of doing harm to our patients. An algorithm would have been tried and tested against thousands of patients, and hence its widespread acceptance, whereas a single physician may have only treated hundreds of patients at most. How could we be entrusted to follow our instincts?

"I reconcile this quandary by asking you to be knowledgeable, thoughtful, to understand pathophysiology, mechanisms of action, and understand the limits of knowledge. Randomized controlled trials, evidence-based medicine, they are gold standards, but they're still imperfect. In many of the meta-analyses, we try to negate the variables of divergent demographics, but there are still issues when you're dealing with the unique person in front of you. Keep in mind, different authoritative bodies may issue differing algorithms or guidelines regarding the same condition."

At this stage, he straightens his back and looks us in the eye. He adopts a stricter tone. This was important.

"*You should be more worried about your patient than you are about the questions which might arise regarding your care.* If you have logical rationale for your actions, you should pursue that approach, even though an algorithm may tell you otherwise. Document why you've taken this course of action. You may be questioned, but you will not be scolded unless your rationale is baseless. But if you say, '*I'm going to follow an algorithm without thinking about it because I'm afraid of what's going to happen in conference if people question me*', then that tells me that you don't have confidence in your understanding of the disease process, or in the treatment options available. If all you can do is follow an algorithm, so can AI.[22] *You're no longer needed, doctor. Very well.*" He thumps the table with his fist, as he portends the demise of the medical profession if we let algorithms and AI hold sway over us. If we allow ourselves to be satisfied with mediocrity. "But if you have that capacity to practice the Art of Infectious Diseases, to use your knowledge of host-pathogen interactions and pharmacology to assess all options, then you will be of benefit to your patient."

But there is the practical side of things; he does acknowledge the need for some leeway in following guidelines and algorithms to the letter. "I totally understand that from the point of view of a trainee though. They are worried because their future is at stake. They are evaluated by their literacy of the ID orthodoxy. '*I've got to take an exam*'. '*I'm being judged by my seniors to determine whether I'm capable or not*'. I understand that. I've lived that experience. But our trainees are extraordinarily gifted, very smart, and have the capacity to think and not just accumulate facts. Once they have acquired fluency with the fundamentals, we should challenge them to creatively solve clinical problems for which there are no convenient solutions."

He closes. "I'm a big fan of algorithms, but I'm always wary of anything being considered perfect or ideal. Everything should be looked at with a certain amount of, not scepticism, but wariness about its applicability in all circumstances." This could be in the form of guidelines, algorithms, artificial intelligence, and most importantly, human intelligence. "As a trainee, you learn from each consultant's knowledge and style of practice. There are take-aways trainees can glean from their work with consultants that's useful to pass exams, but also to practice as an Infectious Diseases physician. Not all consultants are nimble and nuanced in their approach to patient care. But it is to be expected. Different personalities deal with the pressure and uncertainty of patient care in different ways. Just because there are guidelines doesn't mean that attendings will approach cases identically. So we should encourage trainees to ask, '*Why are you doing this differently? What is your rationale?*' Doing so gives the consultant the opportunity to share their insights and wisdom if they haven't already done so."

We remind him that it is not really in our nature to question our teachers or mentors, and he reiterates to us his pet peeve. "One of the first observations I made when I moved to Singapore was that, at least at that time, there was much more formality in the dynamic between the consultant levels and the junior levels. At the time, I thought it might be good operationally, but I hoped that the structure wouldn't interfere with communication."

An aspect of the pandemic that contributed to its complexity for the medical profession was the sheer volume of scientific publications coming out in medical journals, some of which contradicted each other. In one week, remdesivir, an anti-viral drug used to treat COVID-19 patients was shown to have no benefit beyond reducing the length of a patient's hospital stay. In another week, another publication would show that it had no proven benefit at all. Just as the dust started to settle, another publication would state that administering it would reduce a patient's risk of dying from the illness.[23] How was one supposed to form any meaningful policy or give guidance with this?

He reassures us. "That's been the case throughout my professional career. Steroids for alcoholic hepatitis, no steroids for alcoholic hepatitis, nuanced use of steroids for alcoholic hepatitis. It is a given that there is going to be contradiction, overlap, inconsistencies, uncertainties. That's the beauty. As time has passed, the questions have become more refined. Some of the big questions we have a better grasp on, but the nuances we still may not have a grasp on. That does not make me uncomfortable. What it tells us is performing meaningful clinical trials is messy and can be hard. I'm okay with the untidiness and the messiness as long as we take '*givens*' and '*it has been unequivocally proven*' with a grain of salt."

One of the things that happened during the pandemic was the added responsibilities patients had in the management of their health. For the first time, there was a simple-to-use test kit, not related to pregnancy testing, that was easily available to all members of the public. The SARS-CoV-2 antigen rapid test was delivered to all Singaporean households so that its members could diagnose and isolate themselves, or seek medical treatment, should they test positive. The primary intent of this was for public health purposes — easy access to diagnostics allowed for earlier recognition of the illness, and contacts of those infected could self-quarantine earlier, thus limiting the spread in the community. The downside of this was the deluge of patients seeking healthcare, rightfully or not, and demanding treatment. COVID-19 had affected the national psyche and placed the population in a state of perpetual trepidation, and having easy access to diagnostics rendered the healthcare services no favours. In the past, symptoms of COVID-19 would mostly have been brushed off as having a cold or the flu, and if it was mild enough, most would have gone on with their daily lives, or taken sick leave if they were slightly worse for the wear. Now, they presented to doctors informing them that they had COVID-19, which would have posited an anchoring bias in the doctor's assessment right from the get go. What were David's thoughts on how the pandemic had placed health management back, at least partially, into the hands of the patient?

"Health literacy is important. Whatever country you're in, more health literacy is needed. No country has a totally health-literate population. It helps for residents to understand what their obligations are as health care seekers, and what our obligations are as healthcare providers. People have come to me and said, '*I need a CT*[24] *scan*' when they did not have an indication for a CT but needed a different intervention. I would be violating my oath to them to arrange for a CT scan as it's not the appropriate evaluation, and there's a finite risk of malignancy down the road with one.

I inform them that I won't arrange for a CT and why I'm not, but I do recommend a more appropriate next step. I worry that public relations concerns — that we're worried that if we have an unhappy patient, they'll report to some authority that then asks us to explain — unduly impacts patient management and resource utilization."

It certainly weighed heavily on ours. One thing about David is that, often when he comes across one of us who is dealing with a difficult patient or family, he would hear us out, and then willingly offer the gravitas of a senior, White professor to quell any disgruntled families. We were always grateful for that. How had he approached such a situation during his formative years?

"Through observation and serving frequently as a medical expert in medico-legal disputes, I became educated as to what actions result in medical lawsuits and how doctors can decrease the risk of a lawsuit and/or defend themselves if one were to arise. It is not by practising defensive medicine. It isn't by ordering unnecessary tests. It is simply being mindful to provide good care combined with good communication and relevant documentation. I worked on my own listening and communications skills to ensure that I understood what was being asked, and that I answer questions without hyperbole or defensiveness. I've taken this approach not as a public relation effort or from a '*covering my backside*' perspective, but just making sure I understood what the patient's or family's concerns were, to address those concerns with them openly, and to document what I'm doing and why I'm doing it. Not in a 30-page essay, but clearly explaining why I'm doing what I'm doing, and what I have explained. I have received threatening letters from lawyers in the United States, but they were just fishing expeditions. This is a strategy that malpractice attorneys in the US employ to see if they can shake money free without having to litigate. Nothing happens after that. So, my response is — do the right thing medically and equally importantly, you must directly and succinctly address the concern in your documentation…and not via cut and paste."

"This could be challenging in Singapore, because of time constraints and the volume of patients. So with my SRs, I review their notes to determine, '*Have they educated the referring team?*'. Instead of just saying,

'*Stop this antibiotic*', we should say '*We're stopping because we believe the data set is not supportive of an active infection*'. That educates the referring team, and potentially avoids a follow-up message to the ID SR from the team, '*But the consultant wants to continue*'. Additionally, by documenting clearly, someone in the future who is looking at the case can understand your rationale instead of assuming why you took the management course you did. Also, without documentation you may not remember why you did what you did, if a lawsuit comes years later."

He offers some consolation to the junior doctors and healthcare workers who might otherwise be bearing the brunt of a patient's or their family members' wrath. "You cannot control other people. And I know patients and families have been upset with me, and oftentimes I have no earthly idea why despite efforts to understand. Their dissatisfaction may be an expression of their frustration, their fear, of their sense of impotence to change the course of their or their loved one's illness. I can educate, I can empathize. Some things we cannot fix. I've accepted the value of my role as the recipient of their expressions of fear, frustration and sense of powerlessness. The Hippocratic Oath was revised in 1964 to include, '*I will remember that there is art to medicine as well as science, and that warmth, sympathy, and understanding may outweigh the surgeon's knife or the chemist's drug*'. I took that oath and try to adhere to it."

Another way in which the pandemic has changed the way we practiced Medicine is the use of tele-consults. On one hand, it was a boon for the patients — they did not need to travel all the way to the hospital and wait for hours for their consult and their medications. They could be seen by the doctor in the comfort of their home, and have the latter be delivered to their doorstep. On the other hand, it was a bane for patients, and even doctors, who found technology all a little too fiddly, a touch too impersonal, and in truth, a little disconcerting. Which side of the fence did David sit on?

"I already worry about phone consults because there's data to suggest that approximately 40–50% of the information you're told over the phone is incorrect. As such, I'm uncomfortable with virtual *initial* tele-consults. From my limited experience they are not equivalent to face-to-face evaluations when addressing some infectious diseases concerns."

It does seem as though that this was an inevitable road we were headed down.

"I don't know that I'm the right person to speak about tele-consultation, with my limited experience in the States, and to an even lesser degree in Singapore. When I'm providing a tele-consultation, I'm constantly assessing my level of comfort with the appropriateness of remote care for this patient. If I feel that what I'm providing is less than what it should be, then I arrange to see them in person."

"There's a certain amount of physical, non-verbal communication and diagnostic information gained through a physician's trained senses, other than taste, that goes on in a face-to-face consultation that cannot be gleaned from a telemedicine consultation. That said, once I've seen a patient on a first visit and have a better idea of what is occurring, I'm more comfortable with tele-management. But it's that initial process that I'm not comfortable with."

"I recognise we do not have capacity, personnel, space, or time, to see everyone who needs to be seen in person, so alternatives are required. I fully support telemedicine measures. But again, the same mindset — let's be wary and anxious; let's not pat ourselves on the back that we've solved the problem. We should think, '*Is this something you would advocate if the patient was your family member?*'"

For those who might otherwise resist change and hark back on the good old times, he had this to say. "As a registered Singaporean doctor, you took a modified Hippocratic oath. If you feel you are compromising patient care, you're violating your oath. However, I'm trying to be open minded and identify the circumstances I am comfortable providing tele-consultation."

COVID-19 had taken up the bulk of our discussion thus far, but we had one last point to cover. Prof Hsu Li Yang, in '*The Pandemic Cookbook*', said — '*I don't have any particular hopes for the future. We tend to forget things. Most of us have already forgotten the lives lost to get us to this point. And maybe even the CB [circuit breaker] and other events have kind of faded. Those calling for preparedness will be more and more like prophets in the wilderness.*'[25] Did David agree with that pessimistic outlook?

"Is Li Yang being pessimistic or realistic? We repeat history. He's predicting we're going to make the same mistakes we've made before. What is it that is different that will prevent us from doing this? Pandemic preparedness might. If you're going to be comprehensive in pandemic preparedness, it's going to cost an enormous amount, which most countries do not believe they can afford. Has COVID-19 cost trillions of dollars to international GDP?[26] Yes, it has. Pandemic preparedness — how much would it cost? Probably tens of billions as opposed to the trillions we've lost because of COVID-19. A small fraction. But it's tens of billions that countries may not have, or that would otherwise be spent on infrastructure such as schools. Investing in pandemic preparedness, whose work is often not visible to the public, is unlikely to get a politician re-elected. But investing in roads, schools, transportation, et cetera, which are visible and essential for day-to-day living, will. It's not just politics, but it's the cold-blooded necessities of day-to-day governance, and what a society's pressing needs are. How much can you invest for a future, hard-to-predict pandemic when you have needs today? But I think investing in pandemic preparedness is worth the cost. It won't prevent the next pandemic, but I am confident it will mitigate. I understand Li Yang's sentiment, but I am more hopeful that the prophets of doom are being heard — at least for the next few funding cycles."

An important aspect of pandemic preparedness is discussed in the book by Prof Hsu Li Yang and Prof Loh Kah Seng, '*Pandemics in Singapore, 1819–2022*'. In it they state — '*Social memory is a key resource in preparing for the next pandemic, because a pandemic response succeeds only if people recognise that threat.*'[21] To David, ID physicians had to be the lodestar for future pandemics — this was how we remained relevant.

"A major hurdle faced throughout the world was the finite number of isolation facilities. In Singapore, we didn't have enough single rooms to put patients in as cases increased. But we also found, especially early in the pandemic, when we kept people hospitalized in single rooms until their PCRs turned negative, that isolation had dramatic negative economic, psychiatric, educational, and social impacts. Nowadays, we're building more hospitals — not because of COVID-19, but due to increased demand associated with an ageing society. But should those hospitals contain only single rooms as most new builds in Europe and the US do? One of the arguments for single rooms is for Infection Prevention and Control purposes — including preventing or limiting the spread of airborne pathogens. Arguments against single rooms include cost, less efficient use of limited land space, the psychosocial impact of being alone, and so on. I'm confident Infectious Diseases physicians, Infection Prevention and Control professionals, Public Health officials and Health Economists are actively involved in conversations regarding the planning, design and workflows of the new public health institutions being built in Singapore."

In his opinion, what were some of the inexorable changes that COVID-19 has brought about?

"A renewed sense of humility, despite advancements in understanding, diagnostics and care. A reminder that whether we like it or not, the global community is inextricably linked. That *nations must work together* is not a feel-good aspiration but a pragmatic requirement."

At this stage, David signals for a pause. We had run him ragged. He conjures up a 1.5 litre bottle of Coke Zero from his bag and plonks it down on the table in front of us.

"I hope you all aren't offended by me drinking from the tap. And me dissolving my bones in front of your eyes."

We chuckle, after what had been a particularly gruelling discourse. We do not begrudge him, and he proceeds to guzzle down some much-needed tonic.

We move on to the topic of plagues on the horizon, and how we, as ID physicians, could find relevance. A worthwhile quote to note is one by Dr Anthony Fauci, one of the most renowned Infectious Diseases physicians of our times. In his farewell note penned in the NEJM, and in direct contradiction to Dr Robert Petersdorf, he writes, '*When it comes to emerging infectious disease, it's never over…As infectious-disease specialists, we must be perpetually prepared and able to respond to the perpetual challenge.*'[27] It would be foolhardy to presume that David had all the answers to the potential problems plaguing ID, but we wanted him to share the insights he had on the multiple fronts we were set to grapple with.

We begin with not so much an emerging infectious disease, but an emergency in Infectious Diseases — antimicrobial resistance (AMR). Sir Alexander Fleming, discoverer of the antibiotic, penicillin, presciently noted in his Nobel Lecture back in 1945, '*It is not difficult to make microbes resistant to penicillin in the laboratory by exposing them to concentrations not sufficient to kill them, and the same thing has occasionally happened in the body. The time may come when penicillin can be bought by anyone in the shops. Then there is the danger that the ignorant man may easily underdose himself and by exposing his microbes to non-lethal quantities of the drug make them resistant.*'[28] We have spoken about AMR before in Chapter 2, where essentially, the rise of resistance to antimicrobials was all a matter of evolutionary selection pressure on a pathogen. You wouldn't expect German philosophy to have any ties with AMR but it was Friedrich Nietzsche who aptly coined the phrase, '*That which does not kill us makes us stronger*'. Bacteria and other pathogens have existed on this planet long before humans have, and will likely continue to do so long after we are gone. Antimicrobials was just another obstacle for them to overcome. Misuse and overuse of antimicrobials, whether in healthcare or agriculture, are the drivers of AMR. Antimicrobials are the foundation on which modern medicine is built upon, and whether it be surgery or solid organ or bone marrow transplantation, all these will collapse without it. Up to 5 million deaths per year are associated with AMR.[29] As a comparison, global deaths from tuberculosis reached 1.3 million in 2022,[30] and HIV/AIDS-related deaths were a 'mere' 630,000.[31] We were now on the cusp of a post-antimicrobial world. This was serious.

Before we go all doom and gloom, we ask David to comment on a phrase frequently uttered by healthcare professionals — '*Make sure you finish your course of antibiotics or else the bacteria will become resistant.*' Was this message being abused?

"This is a public service campaign, right? That's what that is."

Did he subscribe to it?

"It depends on the infection. But we need consistency in the messaging because people will hear inconsistency if we are not careful with our message. From a public service perspective, you need concrete messaging such as '*finishing your course of antibiotic*', even though as an antibiotic steward you may not agree with the duration, dose or indication for which they were prescribed by the clinician 100% of the time."

"But in the privacy of a clinic with a patient, and the patient is self-flagellating because they only took six days as opposed to seven, I tell them, '*It's okay*'. But that's in the interpersonal dynamic of the office. But I think in general the public service message you quote serves its purpose."

Has he 'intimidated' his patients with this phrase before?

"Yes, a few. I've implored those with fungemia on fluconazole [an antifungal], '*Please just complete your 14 days. It's possible that we'll have an issue if you don't complete it.*' I don't think I've said it for a urinary tract infection, nor a community acquired pneumonia."

How about this other phrase — '*No one should die without meropenem.*' This was a broad-spectrum antibiotic that was typically employed by physicians as a last line of therapy against multi-drug resistant organisms. In our current practice, when patients are suspected to have an infection and are not responding to the commonly prescribed antibiotics, empirical antibiotics are quickly escalated to those with the broadest coverage, for fear of missing out on the treatment of a potentially drug-resistant organism. What were his thoughts on this?

"When employing 'spiralling empiricism' as our antibiotic strategy, we only occasionally or belatedly realise we are in an echo-chamber of our own making. '*The patient will improve if only I find the right antibiotic*'. Rationally, we assess the facts and recognise that the process is not due to an infection, or that a source needs to be drained, or that the antibiotics are the cause of the fever, et cetera. But it can be difficult to allow ourselves to see the bigger picture and break the spiral. Antibiotics are unsatisfying and dangerous as diagnostic tools. We should apply them in that fashion sparingly regardless of which antibiotic we're discussing."

How does one even attempt to draw the line in the use of such broad-spectrum antibiotics?

"The job of an ID physician is to be rational and not succumb to magical thinking or fear, including '*kiasu*-ism.' What a reasonable ID physician would recommend when confronted by the same set of circumstances should be a foundational thought. Reminding ourselves of the unintentional but real harm we can cause with irrational antibiotic use provides perspective to assure sound decision making." Antibiotics, just like any medicinal drug, can have devastating consequences on our patients. It can directly damage the kidneys or the liver, or it can lower the blood cells by suppressing bone marrow function, or it can wipe out the protective bacteria in the gut and have it replaced by a virulent, diarrhoeagenic one — *Clostridioides difficile.*

Back to AMR — what could be done?

"As long as we have an interconnected world, AMR will be a problem — we'll never put the genie back into the bottle. A coordinated approach is required to mitigate the pace of AMR. We don't have infinite resources, so our interventions need to be strategic and synergistic. If we had fewer transmission opportunities, along with alternative therapies, antibiotic stewardship, policies regarding animal and agricultural use, and more incentives for investment in drug development, then maybe that would help."

So, were we doomed?

"I'm optimistic that we can make a difference. What role will bacteriophages, small peptides, antisense or interfering RNA[32] have in the future? I don't know that there will be a tectonic shift in our addressing the problem, but I think we will incrementally have an impact — on at least slowing the pace of AMR spread. Policies, practices and research dollars are being deployed locally and internationally to confront AMR. I'm not confident these efforts will reverse the global trend in the long term."

Climate change is also another problem that we have to contend with. Beyond the direct, devastating effects of extreme temperatures and flooding on the human population, global warming is also predicted to lead to increases in infectious diseases afflicting all life on this planet. As temperate climes warm, geographical coverage of certain vectors such as mosquitoes and ticks expand beyond tropical regions, along with the diseases which are borne on them such as dengue and malaria.[33] Even fungi such as *Coccidioides*, which causes Valley fever and is typically found in the soil in hot and dry areas, have spread from the American Southwest to the Pacific Northwest as a result of climate change and increasing desertification of once fertile land.[34] Whether through droughts or flooding, a rise in waterborne diseases such as cholera or typhoid will ravage vulnerable populations.[35]

As mankind continues to consume the land and our resources irresponsibly, we will be increasingly at risk to novel pathogens carried on wildlife as they invade and adapt to human environments. Locally in Southeast Asia, the then newly discovered pathogen, Nipah virus, afflicted both men and swine in an outbreak between 1998 and 1999. Ironically, humans had a direct hand in bringing about this plague upon ourselves. The fire and haze in Kalimantan, Indonesia, brought about by the slash-and-burn tactics of farming cash craps, forced the horseshoe bats out of the tropical rainforests and into the backyard of humans, the fruit orchards in Kampung Sungai Nipah (Nipah River village). Virus particles from the bat's saliva infected pigs in nearby farms, as the latter consumed the half-eaten fruits left behind by the former, thus facilitating the cross-species jump by the virus. Another cross-species leap was then made as the virus infected humans through direct contact or consumption of infected animals and their body fluids, and a deadly outbreak ensued.[36] Singapore was not unscathed either. Pigs from an affected farm in Malaysia were imported onto the island, and this subsequently caused an outbreak amongst abattoir workers. Eleven men were affected, with a single fatality.[37] Human's continued disruption of nature will continually put us at risk of such emerging infectious diseases. Cumulatively, together with the disruption and destruction of existing infrastructure and health systems, and the forced migration of climate refugees which may yet lead to even more contagion, we are on the cusp of a humanitarian crisis and an infectious disease apocalypse.

"Yellow fever and malaria used to be an issue in the States, and dengue is being transmitted sporadically there. I suspect all of these will intermittently arise to varying degrees in their old haunts and so we will have to learn to adapt. It is clear we're going to have more infectious disease as well as non-communicable disease deaths as a consequence of environmental extremes."

Could he still remain optimistic?

"I am an optimist as a consequence of witnessing individuals' passion for change and willingness to press for action on matters important to them. However, moving governments to act generally requires more than passion alone, instead there is more cost-benefit, risk-reward analysis and less emotion. The threshold needed for policy makers to act on issues is either too high or too low for many of us depending on the specific issue: health, education, corruption, or climate change. Policy changes which take place prior to crisis often requires bold and courageous leadership. It is not easy for a leader to say, '*I know there are those of you who don't agree, but we have to do this*', particularly when your position is in the minority."

He refers us back to our current predicament. "We saw that during COVID-19, right? It reached a bar where countries hurt themselves before they could help themselves." An example of this was the United Kingdom, where a lack of leadership allowed the virus to spread exponentially through the country and devastate the population. Ironically, this allowed them to be at the forefront of clinical research and some of the important COVID-19 therapeutic measures, such as the life-saving use of steroids in critically ill patients, arose from this.

"With climate change, I don't know how a major step forward in addressing the issue is going to happen. Because to achieve that change, like with COVID-19, it will require cooperation across nations. I'm less optimistic that geopolitical powers can effectively work together in a meaningful and timely fashion. Governments are transactional and not typically altruistic when dealing with each other." This was a rare occasion where the glass was half empty for David.

People with vaccine hesitancy, or more crudely known as 'anti-vaxxers', were a particular vexation for the ID community during the COVID-19 pandemic. It was a plague we had to deal with on a second front, when we were already swamped with the first. But it was not a new phenomenon, having already existed since the first vaccine was introduced back in the 19th century.[38] Crucially, we did not help ourselves when one of our own falsely linked autism with the MMR[39] vaccine, back in 2008.[40] Measles, a disease earmarked for extinction, rebounded in the community and led to innumerable hospitalizations and even to a couple of deaths. This has carried on into the new millennia and all throughout the pandemic, and even tore families apart.[41] What does an ID physician need to do to convert the unbelievers?

"ID physicians can be more visible. We can speak up more, earnestly, honestly, and not be a chest thumper or a hyperbolic carnival hack. The ID community has not tried to outshout the anti-vaxxers, but it is sometimes hard to be heard above the din. We tend to keep our head down and beaver away in the background. As long as we're science-based, and we're open about the limits of science, and acknowledge that this is what we know today, that we sincerely believe this to be the right thing, then our message will be heard. We should acknowledge that our recommendations may change tomorrow. We adapt to that change. That's how care evolves — it is not linear." This was all rather optimistic, but he was encouraging us to remain as humble and as honest as possible when dealing with the anti-science brigade.

"And that's why I'm keen for motivated, capable ID-trained physicians to look beyond clinical practice and see other opportunities to share the perspectives they have gained from ID training. Become a politician, policymaker, researcher, run a biotech company, teach, et cetera. Your voice matters. We will have enough people to manage clinical infectious diseases. Go out from the comfortable confines of the public health institution where you've gained your knowledge and be all you can be." He pauses there for a while and frowns momentarily. And then he adds. "I hate to quote the US Army enrolment campaign phrase."[42]

It may be all too soon, but what did he think the next pandemic might be?

"Well, I don't have a crystal ball, but it's likely influenza or coronavirus. To provide perspective, while pandemics justifiably focus our attention, we live in a world where there're lots of potentially preventable lethal items we should be aware of, whether it's environmental, microbiological, trauma, obesity, et cetera."

We had spoken quite a lot about the potential plagues that ensured our jobs as ID physicians, but now, we wanted to touch on one other that could potentially make us irrelevant. Artificial intelligence. It is the in-thing now, especially with the arrival of large language models, heralded by ChatGPT.[43] We'd briefly touched on it earlier on in the session, but we wanted to discuss more about it in depth. What were his thoughts on AI-led medicine?

"I really wouldn't worry. Patients need human interaction from their healer. There are shamanistic undertones to what we do. No one wants to die with AI managing them. The frailties of being a human being, the issues of end of life or birth or critical diagnosis are not just physical experiences, they're emotional experiences. You can't provide that with AI…yet. They [the patients] need us."

It does sound as though we were relegated back to offering moral support whilst losing our critical thinking.

"I'm not suggesting you defer to AI to make the diagnosis and the management plan and then we'll just hold our patient's hand. If you think about it, even now, we use databases and our experience when we see patients. We refer to various databases and algorithms to provide content and suggested and/or evidence-based approaches. AI is a similar process, but on steroids — a lot more data and more refined analytical capacity. AI is limited by the biases in the data it accesses, its solution solving limited to its algorithms and their biases, and at least for the time being, a lack of transference. And so, I don't see us disappearing because I don't see there being perfect bias-free databases and algorithms that negate my capacity to value add."

We counter. This database from AI is going to be worldwide. It's going to have more knowledge than any of us can accrue. Is that not what is best for our patients?

"AI doesn't say to the patient, '*What is it that you want? What's of value to you? What matters? What is it your family wants? Let me share with you the implications of what is being prioritised by AI.*' What they [the patients] want to hear is, '*I have reviewed and made an analysis of your circumstances, and suggest that we do this, after having spoken with you, and understanding what's important to you. This plan of action is the best option to meet your personal needs compared to all the other options available.*' That's what patients want. They don't need a printout. They need someone to be an interface between the crunching of databases, the analysis of data, the generation of a course of action, and themselves. I still think they need a human being to be able to put all of it into context. We can interpret what AI is suggesting to assure it a person-specific experience. We are needed to refine AI's algorithms. AI will play a greater role, but I don't know that we're ever going away." To him, AI was just another tool in the bag. It will revolutionise humanity, just like fire had, just like the wheel had, just like the combustion engine had, just like the internet had. But we were always in control, and never overwhelmed. We could not be made irrelevant with such blunt tools. AI seemed different though, but David wasn't convinced that we, doctors, could ever be replaced. We just needed to make sure that we didn't allow it to dull our senses.

We're back to square one now, to an age-old question. We've seen the plagues that existed, that exist, and that will come to exist. Their presence ensures our relevance as a specialty. But one thing that has always plagued our minds was job security. This could apply to just about any specialty, but we have on average five to six Infectious Diseases specialists joining the fold annually, and in a decade, that can amount to quite a significant number. We revisit what Dr Robert Petersdorf said again — were we going to be spending time culturing one another, or was there still more room on the agar plate?

"I'm not concerned about too many ID physicians. It is great for Singapore medicine and Singaporeans in general. There will be ID trainees who successfully exit their exams and have concerns regarding what and where they will work. But there'll always be opportunities. The more qualified ID physicians we have, the more we raise the ID literacy of the community. Some ID physicians may not end up practicing ID. They may become primary care physicians. I don't see that as a wasted opportunity or a bad thing. I'm familiar with many successful, happy ID-trained physicians outside of Singapore who work as primary care physicians with ID expertise. I also hope someday that HIV care is not centralized, that it can be managed by HIV-literate physicians, whether they are ID-trained or not, in the community. I am aware that this is not a popular notion or logistically feasible in the current environment. I'm not naive. I'm not seeking a revolution, but it would be a step in the direction of normalizing HIV and impacting the stigma associated with HIV."

One of the arguments put forward by junior doctors in Singapore was that — if there weren't going to be jobs for them after completing training, why accept them into training in the first place, only to languish after that?

"As unpopular as this may sound, it's not the ID-training Programme Director's job to assure a job is waiting for an applicant at the end of their training. Employment assurance at the end of training may have been explicitly stated or implied in the past, but it is not the current practice in Singapore. It's the training programme's job to provide a trainee with the means to become a qualified ID physician, the opportunities to explore their interests in the field of ID, and hopefully identify a niche for themselves; thus, making themselves attractive as an employee or partner to institutions, companies, or practices with a need for their skillset. So as unsettling as that may sound, and maybe because my career path has been atypical, being well-trained and encouraged to explore their opportunities will result in the best possible outcome for all involved. Capable people, and this describes the trainees accepted into Singapore ID-training programmes, will adapt, adjust and find a way to be professionally productive and happy."

He throws the ball back into our court. "As ID physicians we need to guard against resting on our laurels once we have our speciality certification. That recognition need not be our final professional goal. We should allow ourselves to imagine beyond the traditional roles that ID physicians assume: clinician, administrator, teacher or researcher." These were the typical key performance indicators that a doctor in the public sector was assessed by — their output in relation to their clinical, research, educational and administrative work. But David was advocating for us to be more than that. To not allow ourselves to be pigeon-holed. Just like how he had refused to conform all those years back. "We should also be policy makers, advisors, members of think tanks, or politicians. Our hard-earned, analytical skills are transferrable to other fields such as finance and IT. Think outside the box." In other words, be all we could be. The world was our oyster.

To the up-and-coming ID trainees, even covert ones, he had this to say. "Focus on the joy of learning this wonderful area of Medicine [ID]. It is so fascinating. It forces us to witness what it is to be human, to be mortal, joyous, frightened, and alive. It is ever revealing new secrets. It forces us to learn even if we are not inclined."

David wasn't defined by being just an ID physician alone. He was more than that, and he wanted us to realise that we could be more than that too. ID was just one facet of life, a set of skills that could find utility in its many other aspects. We could not and should not let it limit our potential and our imagination. This was the point he was trying to get across. As Dr Anthony Fauci succinctly puts it, '*The mosaic of your knowledge and experiences is eternally unfinished, as it should be.*'

He brings things to a close by recognising its true value. "You're a better person because of it. You're a better doctor because of it. Those are good things. These benefits make the journey all the more worthwhile."

We shouldn't allow ID to plague us down.

Notes

1   H. Kelsey. 'Pestilence and playwright', *Shakespeare birthplace trust.* Shakespeare Birthplace Trust. 7 Sep 2016. [https://www.shakespeare.org.uk/explore-shakespeare/blogs/pestilence-and-playwright/]

2   J Kennedy. (2023) 'Pathogenesis: How germs made history'. Torva.

3   Severe acute respiratory syndrome coronavirus 2

4   Severe acute respiratory syndrome caused by the original SARS-CoV

5   Middle East respiratory syndrome caused by the Middle East respiratory syndrome coronavirus (MERS-CoV)

6   A public health terminology meaning to spread out the rate of infections so as not to overwhelm vital healthcare systems and infrastructure

7   To be pedantic, the term 'quarantine' is utilised when contacts of an infected personnel are segregated from the general population for the period of incubation of the infectious agent [2-14 days for SARS-CoV-2], whether or not they have been infected. The term 'isolation' is utilised when an infected person is segregated from the general population for the period of their infectiousness [typically 2 days before symptoms onset for COVID-19, and up to 10 days thereafter].

8   WHO COVID-19 dashboard. WHO. [https://covid19.who.int/] (accessed 31 Jan 2024)

9   W. J. Abdullah. 'Singapore's Responses to the COVID-19 Outbreak: A Critical Assessment', *The American Review of Public Administration.* 2020 50(6–7), 770–776.

10   'The Fauci Phenomenon', *N Engl J Med.* 2023 Mar 9;388(10):e28.

11   Singapore's version of a lockdown

12   PM Lee: the COVID-19 situation in Singapore. gov.sg. 3 Apr 2020. [https://www.gov.sg/article/pm-lee-hsien-loong-on-the-covid-19-situation-in-singapore-3-apr]

13   Trump suggests US slow virus testing to avoid bad statistics. AP News. 21 Jun 2020. [https://apnews.com/article/virus-outbreak-donald-trump-ap-top-news-joe-biden-tulsa-476068bd60e9048303b736e9d7fc6572]

14   Trump directs experts to see whether they can bring 'light inside the body' to kill the coronavirus, even as his own expert shuts him down. Business Insider. 24 Apr 2020. [https://www.businessinsider.com/trump-wants-bring-light-inside-the-body-to-kill-coronavirus-2020-4]

[15] WHO impressed by how Singapore handles coronavirus outbreak. The Straits Times. 20 Feb 2020. [https://www.straitstimes.com/singapore/who-impressed-by-how-spore-handles-outbreak]

[16] From Singapore to the World: Where Fortitude Kit Has Been Deployed Globally. A*STAR. 27 Mar 2020. [https://www.a-star.edu.sg/News/astarNews/news/covid-19/from-singapore-to-the-world-where-fortitude-kit-has-been-deployed-globally]

[17] NUS invents new way to produce Covid-19 swab, 40 million to be produced in coming months. The Straits Times. 13 Jul 2020. [https://www.straitstimes.com/singapore/health/nus-invents-new-way-to-produce-covid-19-swab-40-million-to-be-produced-in-coming]

[18] COVID-19: Shedding light on the plight and laws regulating migrant worker dormitories in Singapore. NUS Law. [https://law.nus.edu.sg/impact/covid-19-shedding-light-on-the-plight-and-laws-regulating-migrant-worker-dormitories-in-singapore/] (accessed 31 Jan 2024)

[19] Permanent resident

[20] Emergency Department

[21] K. S. Loh and L. Y. Hsu. (2023) 'Pandemics in Singapore, 1819–2022 (Routledge Studies in the Modern History of Asia)'. Routledge.

[22] Artificial intelligence

[23] R. C. Maves. 'Making Sense of Contradictory Evidence in Coronavirus Disease 2019 Trials', *Clin Infect Dis*. 2021 Jan 25:ciab012.

[24] Computed tomography

[25] L. Y. Hsu and S. Liew. (2022) 'The Pandemic Cookbook'. Epigram Books.

[26] Gross domestic product

[27] A. S. Fauci. 'It Ain't Over Till It's Over ... but It's Never Over — Emerging and Reemerging Infectious Diseases', *N Engl J Med*. 2022 Dec 1;387(22):2009–2011.

[28] A. Fleming. 'Penicillin', *Nobel Lecture*. 11 Dec 1945. [https://www.nobelprize.org/uploads/2018/06/fleming-lecture.pdf]

[29] 'Vaccines could avert half a million deaths associated with anti-microbial resistance a year'. WHO. 28 Jul 2023. [https://www.who.int/news/item/28-07-2023-vaccines-could-avert-half-a-million-deaths-associated-with-anti-microbial-resistance-a-year]

[30] 'Tuberculosis'. WHO. 7 Nov 2023. [https://www.who.int/news-room/fact-sheets/detail/tuberculosis]

31 UNAIDS. 'Fact Sheet', World AIDS Day 2023. [https://www.unaids.org/sites/default/files/media_asset/UNAIDS_FactSheet_en.pdf]

32 Ribonucleic acid

33 M. C. Thomson and L. R. Stanberry. 'Climate Change and Vectorborne Diseases', *N Engl J Med*. 2022 Nov 24;387(21):1969–1978.

34 An Invisible Killer. The Washington Post. 13 Nov 2023. [https://www.washingtonpost.com/climate-environment/interactive/2023/valley-fever-spread-climate-change-coccidioides-fungus/]

35 J. C. Semenza and A. I. Ko. 'Waterborne Diseases That Are Sensitive to Climate Variability and Climate Change', *N Engl J Med*. 2023 Dec 7;389(23):2175–2187.

36 Nipah: fearsome virus that caught the medical and scientific world off-guard. The Guardian. 18 Jan 2017. [https://www.theguardian.com/world/2017/jan/18/nipah-fearsome-virus-that-caught-the-medical-and-scientific-world-off-guard]

37 N. I. Paton et al. 'Outbreak of Nipah-virus infection among abattoir workers in Singapore', *Lancet*. 1999 Oct 9;354(9186):1253-6.

38 A. Parodi and M. Martini. 'History of vaccine and immunization: Vaccine-hesitancy discussion in Germany in XIX century', *Vaccine*. 2023 Mar 17;41(12):1989–1993.

39 Measles, mumps and rubella

40 The Vaccine-Autism Myth Started 20 Years Ago. Here's Why It Still Endures Today. Time. 28 Feb 2018. [https://time.com/5175704/andrew-wakefield-vaccine-autism/]

41 Families Try Making Up After Pandemic Fights Over Vaccines, Masks and Tests. The Wall Street Journal. 25 Feb 2022. [https://www.wsj.com/articles/families-try-making-up-after-pandemic-fights-over-vaccines-masks-and-tests-11645757654]

42 Be all you can be. 1-800-USA-ARMY

43 Chatbox Generative Pre-trained Transformer

CONSULTATIONS

–

non sibi sed omnibus
'not for oneself but for all'

Why do doctors quit?

To understand why doctors leave the medical profession, you must first understand why they join it. And to that latter question, the answer, if not an over-simplification, is the invariable need to be a hero. If you read the personal statements of medical school hopefuls, the responses more or less centre around a singular truth — they want to help someone. The applicant may have confronted a tragic loss amidst their circle of friends or family, or were themselves experiencing an exacting medical condition, or were drawn by the plight of the poor and the destitute whilst on a mission trip, and hence they aspired to join the medical fraternity to make a difference. There is nothing demeaning in this. It is aspirational. It is altruistic. It is praise-worthy. It is worthy of pursuit. Dr William Osler states, in no uncertain terms — *'The practice of Medicine is an art, not a trade; a calling, not a business; a calling in which your heart will be exercised equally with your head.'* Practicing Medicine was of a higher order; it was a passion that consumed you entirely.

However, what is typically not included in such statements are the hardly obscure but glitzy and glamorous aspects of the profession. Being a doctor comes with a certain prestige. It is one of the most respected professions in the world, simply because of the nature of the work. People from all aspects of life seek out your services, from the incarcerated to the regal, from the cradle to the grave. It is associated with having the smarts, together with a complementary tail of incomprehensible letters extending beyond the name. These are worn like a badge of honour. And there is job security with a stable pay in which one will not be in want. Put in a nutshell, you get paid well doing a noble job, a career that would afford recognition in society.

Yet, and it may be a tad of an overgeneralization but, personal statements are typically written by whippersnappers, young adults or even teenagers still wet behind the ears. In Singapore, unless you are one of the few who study Medicine as a post-graduate degree in the Duke-NUS Medical School, one customarily enters into medical training between the ages of 18 to 19. They would have been fresh out of their years in junior college. They would have had little to no work or life experience. They would not, at that age, truly comprehend what was in store for them. How are they to know what a career for a lifetime truly entails? How can they truly envision how the next 50 to 60 years of their lives will pan out? How are they to know that dreams and priorities change as they hurtle through the different stages of life?

And then it begins, insidiously, during their years in university. The long hours of lectures and tutorials to endure. A deluge of medical texts to get through and memorize after hours. The countless assessments and examinations to navigate through. Three years later, just as they are thick in the throes of their clinical years, their peers in other faculties graduate and begin their careers, finally having some money of their own to spend. But in just another two years, they themselves would be able to join the ranks of their peers. They could stomach that, and they do graduate, eventually. The proudest moment of their lives, up till then. And then the work starts, and the gnawing continues.

The first aspect of their lives that they lose is control of their time — lunchtime belongs to that family who has one too many queries; a dinner engagement with their old clique belongs to that patient who suffers a cardiac arrest on a Friday evening; weekends and public holidays belong to the wards of patients under their team's care, because a hospital has no off days. And then there are the calls, the dreadful overnight hours that happen not too infrequently, where a skeletal crew of doctors man what is akin to a sinking ship, plugging holes and scooping buckets of water out, just to keep it afloat till the cavalry arrives at dawn. The next day, they lumber on in a zombified state, struggling to stay awake till at least noon, when their 36-hour work day ends. Then they're back at work again in less than 24 hours, and the cycle of timelessness repeats. As they progress in their career, there is even more demand placed on their time. Dinner with their children and family is replaced by a tediously long and complicated surgery, so much so that they frequently return home only to see their children asleep. Sleep continues to be disrupted at night as a patient goes into labour at three in the morning and they rush down to clamp the umbilical cord. Anniversary meals with their spouse are a hasty event as they rush to make it on time to deliver that Saturday afternoon lecture. Nights after dinner, and after the children have slept, are spent preparing these very same lectures and tutorials, or keeping up to date with the latest medical literature, or preparing for yet more assessments and examinations in this career of lifelong learning, or worrying about that very patient that they had just operated on. This calling never dies down.

The second aspect of their lives that they lose is their pride. They are surrounded by unreasonableness. The unreasonable patient. The one who threatens to abscond from the hospital in the middle of the night, and verbally abuses the junior doctor on duty to get his way, all because he had been denied discharge by the medical team during the day. The unreasonable patient's family. The ones who demand that the patient be seen only by senior consultants and emeritus professors, who demean the achievements of junior doctors because they are just not adequately qualified in their eyes. The unreasonable senior doctor. The ones who humiliate the juniors by demanding that they improve their standards in medical note-writing, yet themselves do not exhibit the same calibre exacted from their juniors. The unreasonable pressures of the work culture itself. The morning clinic compacted with upwards of thirty patients, with an insufficient five minutes for each to be seen. The only definitive result that follows from this is compromised patient care. The afternoon then follows in the same vein, and the days ahead follow in the same suit. It can all be a little undignified, on top of the inordinate amount of time hampered by electronic documentation, typing up patient notes, discharge summaries, memos, prescriptions, and what nots. Time which could have been spent doing what they had originally signed up for all those years back — caring for patients. Eventually, a shell is all that remains.

In simple terms, they call it a day because of disillusionment.

It is a dire picture that we have painted, but these voices of disaffection and disgruntlement have been growing, and will continue to grow louder over the years. There are problems to address and issues to resolve, undoubtedly, but many of them have no solutions. For those, empathy, inspiration, and encouragement are what is needed. Having inspired many generations of young physicians in the past, we get David to chronicle his experiences and advice for the next and future generations of young physicians, but also not neglecting those still young at heart. This section takes a more introspective turn as we discuss these matters that are close to the hearts of doctors.

Many of us, like the protagonist in '*A Country Doctor's Notebook*'[1] by Mikhail Bulgakov, struggle with the transition from medical school to actual apprenticeship. In the book, Mikhail, a young, newly graduated doctor, flails and flounders as he begins his independent practice in rural Russia. He was an excellent student, but had difficulties grappling with applying theoretical knowledge to actual clinical practice — '*I had perfectly good vision, [but] my eyes [were] as yet unclouded by experience.*' The tension lies between having enough 'head knowledge' which medical school prepares you for, and actual practical 'clinical acumen' or 'clinical decision-making'. Once again, the quote-worthy Dr William Osler had something to say about this — '*He who studies Medicine without books sails an uncharted sea, but he who studies Medicine without patients does not go to sea at all.*' We asked pointedly — how does one deal with the situation when a patient does not agree with the treatment plan but instead chooses a more 'inferior' approach?

David empathizes with this dilemma. "That's a very good question which we deal with not infrequently. Maybe early on in my career, I felt that I had an obligation to force them to see the world my way." Over the years of practice, his youthful, hubristic view about the role of doctors has evolved and matured over time. "But I don't any longer."

He elaborates further. "In such instances, I try to understand why another treatment approach is preferred. Is it due to a lack of trust, cost, fear of consequences, belief system or values, or alternative information? With that understanding, and if they are open to further consideration, I can attempt to address amenable issues. Additionally, addressing a patient's perceived conflict between their values and belief systems and our recommended management plans may benefit from family and/or spiritual assistance."

This last point piqued our interest. Before the advent of modern medicine, health and illness was typically viewed by patients as a spiritual event, and religious belief and practice helped to provide answers. This approach to patient advocacy — seeking religious assistance — was something that we as junior doctors had hardly ever encountered before. We sought out more details.

"Dr Edmund Monteiro and I were seeing a patient who was in need of guidance beyond what his family was able to provide. We consulted a Catholic priest who paid a visit and provided counselling. This happened more than once."

We spoke to both Dr Edmund Monteiro as well as Ms Iris Verghese to find out more about this.[2,3] Ms Verghese was a former public health officer working together with David and Dr Monteiro at the CDC back in the late 1980s to stem the HIV epidemic. Some of the patients had indeed been visited by a religious personnel, but he was not a priest. He was a religious brother — the late Brother Emmanuel. He had been a previous executive director of Boys' Town, and regularly went to the CDC to visit some of those who were under his care, and to provide spiritual counselling.

In a similar vein, we ask David to comment about the issue of non-adherence. Many times, patients keep returning to seek healthcare in a medical crisis, all because they were not taking their pills that were prescribed. This could be disastrous in many ways, with a diabetic coming in with a gangrenous foot that needed to be amputated, or a patient with tuberculosis now coming in with a multi-drug resistant strain that required them to be incarcerated for the duration of their treatment. This was all particularly frustrating for doctors, because it could all have been so easily prevented.

"I will open by saying, patients have autonomy. Patients have values that may align or not with ours. Seek to understand the reasons for non-compliance. Attempt to understand the patient's perspective — are there treatment side-effects, poor comprehension due to issues such as education, cognitive decline, or substance abuse, mental health barriers, loneliness, in addition to those issues mentioned in my response to the prior question. I have an obligation to educate them and to assure they have heard and understood what I am recommending, to be their advocate, to be sure they're making an informed decision. It is not for me to say what is their best life. I respect their wishes. Health is only one part of their life. They live in a community, they have relationships, and they have wants, needs, and desires. My duty is to help them understand and put into context the gravity of their current situation."

Beyond the issues faced by patients on the ground, he highlights the additional barriers that have to be dealt with at a systems level. "There are several hurdles to the current health care delivery system's ability to more comprehensively address non-adherence. Amongst those are fragmentation of healthcare with resultant lack of relationship building, health literacy, and effective communication."

He empathizes with the perennial exasperation experienced by doctors in their dealings with the non-adherent patient, but for that, he urges us to channel our energies into something positive. "Doctor frustration without action is not helpful. We should provide feedback for our observations regarding preventable morbidity and avoidable healthcare costs. Singapore is aware that healthcare delivery needs to expand from excellent and expensive acute care delivery to excellent but ultimately less costly community-based care — screening, prevention, chronic care management, and end of life care. Rethinking what role public health institutions play in a community in addressing all the determinants of health — not just medical — may allow us to deploy our finite resources more effectively, and possibly decrease admissions due to non-compliance or delays in access to chronic care."

Back on a personal level, we quote David a contradictory view from the late Dr Paul Farmer, an Infectious Diseases physician in the US who had passed away in 2022. He was a champion of the poor, and stated in his biography '*Mountains Beyond Mountains*',[4] '*The only non-compliant people are physicians. If the patient doesn't get better, it's your own fault. Fix it.*' Dr Farmer himself used to routinely trek for hours to reach remote villages in Haiti so as to personally administer medication to his patients. To him, the buck stopped with the physician, and one had to do all they could to service their patients. Any negative patient outcome that could have been prevented was essentially the fault of the medical team. Did David agree with the late Dr Farmer's approach to patient advocacy?

"No, not as quoted. Oddly, the message has messianic and patriarchal overtones simultaneously. The approach can be read to have the potential to steamroll patient autonomy. I appreciate the desire, which is to address healthcare inequity, but I would favour an empowerment approach which can be more needs-focused and efficient."

Many junior doctors fear a negative outcome, and are even more fearful that they are the reason for that outcome. How far did our duty of care extend to our patients?

"Our duty of care extends to being attentive, diligent, competent and up to date with our efforts to diagnosis and manage patients. We have a duty to seek out and arrange for competent care if we are not able to due to inexperience or capacity. In carrying out our duty we should not ignore the doctrine of proportionality: the benefits of our efforts should exceed the burden. We have a duty to recognise futility and not allow patient suffering in service to our egos."

He emphasises one final point. "Running your concerns past others and seeking a fresh perspective is never shameful, it's smart — no matter what phase of your career."

What we had just touched upon was about a patient's *autonomy*, one of the four pillars of medical ethics, the right of competent adults to make informed decisions about their own medical care. However, in Singapore, and perhaps other Asian settings, it is a little more complicated than that. The family is seen as the basic unit of society, and there have been many instances where family members are involved in decision-making and corrode or corrupt the patient's own values. This often poses a challenge for junior doctors, as they try to balance the family's wishes against what is perceived to be best for the patient. It is not uncommon to hear from our patients, especially the older ones, to relieve themselves of the burden of decision making by telling their doctors, '*Please ask my children/family members what they think is best for me.*' This occurs even though they have the capacity to make these decisions for themselves. It impedes their care as an additional hurdle needs to be overcome by the medical team contacting a family member to seek approval, and in times of an emergency, it inadvertently becomes a stressful situation. It is unfair on the family member as well, to make potentially difficult decisions on behalf of a loved one. What do we do when family members become embroiled in a patient's care?

This was a culture entirely foreign to David. "I still struggle with that a little bit in Singapore. In the US, it's very clear to me — my obligation is the patient. I took an oath to take care of that patient, not their family. I do follow the patient's explicit directives to me. If they instruct me to take into consideration their family's decisions, or if the patient is unable to participate in decision making, then their next-of-kin serves the role of informing me of their relative's wishes. However, if family intervenes in the care of a capable patient's care without the patient's explicit consent, then I'm obligated to respect the patient's autonomy and I respectfully decline to consider the family's wishes as the final word. In the scenario when family wishes to direct care without the patient's consent, I also keep in mind the possibility that their intentions may have less noble objectives."

His advice to us?

"Try to understand why family members may want to assume that role, and how we as doctors are perceived by the patient and family. The actions of family members are often in response to one or several concerns, including their parent's well-being, cognitive function and capacity to comprehend, which is affected by education, language, and decline; the child's sense of obligation, financial concerns, legal obligation, guilt, fear; and/or family dynamics and values. We may not be aware of these concerns. But what is crucial is that understanding and taking these concerns into consideration may give us insight into finding a solution which provides an opportunity for the patient to exercise his or her autonomy, as appropriate."

At this juncture, he illuminates an important point here that does not often cross our minds. "Those of us caring for the patient in hospital can be perceived by the patient's children as a well-trained and well-intentioned but one-off functionary, thrust into their parent's and her family's life, given the authority to provide life-impacting recommendations for their loved one. Generally, the patient nor family selected us. The relationship is often transactional and superficial — at a minimum, addressing only those needs which require immediate attention. The patient and family typically grant us their trust without being afforded the time nor relationship building process usually required to earn trust. This is a different dynamic than may exist in the outpatient setting, where patients and their doctor can establish a long-term relationship based on mutual understanding and trust."

David, here, was reminding us about the vulnerability of the patient. They are at a disadvantage — physically from their medical condition; and mentally in terms of comprehending their disease trajectory. Their circumstances are not too dissimilar to that of a prisoner trapped in a hostage situation — they have no bargaining power. The confidence afforded to us doctors is, truth be told, no more than a matter of exigency. Thus, though it can be frustrating to have to deal with the 'difficult' patient or family, the sacrosanct relationship between a doctor and his or her patient must not be allowed to be eroded from a lack of accommodation.

One particularly delicate issue that junior doctors often face on the ground is determining the goals of care for a patient, especially when family members, out of a sense of duty and desperation, may demand certain medical interventions that may not truly be in the best interest of the patient. A not too infrequent scenario encountered would be that of the elderly patient with dementia, who is unable to care for him or herself independently, who presents with a medical emergency whereby intensive care is required just to tide over the initial critical phase. This may mean subjecting the patient to multiple invasive lines and intubation, though it is not a guarantee that he or she will survive this particular encounter because of their frailty. Yet the plea invoked by a family member to '*do all you can*' is exceptionally hard to ignore. What runs through David's mind in such instances?

"I would advocate that goals and limits of care should be established for every patient at the time of hospitalisation regardless of their acuity or, even better, during outpatient visits. Asking the patient's wishes on these topics is no different than asking if they've been taking their medication or have new symptoms — it can be addressed matter-of-factly and provide an opening for a deeper exploration. Having these conversations before a crisis serves several purposes. Firstly, it provides patient and family education. Secondly, it provides perspective that all healthcare delivery, or absence of healthcare, carries risk. Thirdly, it demonstrates to the patient the doctor's holistic care, and finally, it normalizes the conversation regarding the human experience. In those situations when patients or families become upset by raising the issues of goals of care and limits of care, I find it provides an opportunity to explore their values and concerns regarding a topic which we must all eventually address one way or another. More often, I've had patients thank me for raising the often-taboo topic. Having a primary caregiver who has earned their patient's trust can de-stress this issue for those so inclined. If we do not address this topic when circumstances are less pressing and less emotionally charged, we do a disservice to patients, their families, and the caregivers charged with their oversight when the patient is hospitalized in distress." In other words, he was a proponent for a proactive rather than reactive stance to such events.

How though, should a junior approach this situation, if such discussions had not been held previously? How does one balance the use of medical resources against sustaining a patient's life?

"If prior discussions regarding goals and limits of care have not taken place and decisions need to be made quickly, then we attempt to learn the patient's, or family's, insight into the condition, expectations, and values. The responses may be impacted by the gravity of the situation and possibly different than if solicited in less fraught times. Honest discussions regarding possible differences between quality of life versus quantity of life, the realities of ICU care, such as isolation, disorientation, possibly uncomfortable procedures, deconditioning, et cetera, in other words, beneficence, non-maleficence, autonomy, and justice, are critical."

On the topic of limited resources, we bring up the medical ethical principle of *justice* and the issue of healthcare efficiency. Every aspect of a patient's stay in hospital is quantifiable — the cost of a test, the cost of a drug, and even the cost per day of a patient's inpatient hospital stay.

This was the economics of healthcare, and every professional is expected to practice healthcare equitably in this day and age. Invariably, it is very different when there is a patient in front of you. Case in point, there may be a bedbound patient under your care who is awaiting a non-urgent scan that can only happen four days later, yet is clinically well enough to be discharged first. You would save cost by discharging the patient home first, and also free up space for a new admission. Yet, this would incur a lot of hassle and cost to the patient and their family members to arrange another trip down to the hospital on another day, whether in the form of transport, or having to take time off from work. Had efficiency become a bane rather than a boon for patients?

He deliberates for a bit before replying. "This is a matter of public education, policy and politics. What is the role of the hospital in a healthcare delivery model, especially with regards to efficient resource utilization, logistics and prioritization? I think we need medical economists to provide feedback as to whether or not those actions we do in the name of efficiency truly deliver...and we, as patient advocates, need to make an assessment at what 'cost' is that efficiency gained." However, with the patient in front of him, there were no two ways about it. "It's my job to be an advocate for my patient. If I think their condition is life-threatening or the 'efficient approach' is going to compromise their health in a significant way, I will manage the patient in a manner as most appropriate for their well-being."

Since junior doctors are not trained medical economists, how would he advise them to think about medical equity whilst advocating for the patient in front of them?

"The doctor's primary duty in Singapore is to the patient. The SMC's Physician Pledge states — '*make the health of my patient my first consideration*'. Health is defined by the WHO since the 1940s as — '*Health is a state of complete physical, mental and social well-being and not merely the absence of disease or infirmity.*' My advice is to understand the complete meaning and obligations of the pledge, apply that to the patient's circumstances and take a just course of action."

At the start of our careers as doctors, psychological tensions often build up in the care of our patients, and we struggle with these, and often find it hard to let go. Mikhail Bulgakov goes on to mention, in '*A Country*

Doctor's Notebook', that it was a challenge to be *'calm and cautious yet at the same time utterly decisive and unfaltering'*. It is often a heavy burden, especially in this current medical climate, to balance being firm in a clinical decision, and yet having very little room to make mistakes. We deal with patients and family members who can search for 'answers' to their ailment on the internet, and barrage us with an infinite number of queries; and we also deal with patients who are trigger happy and post on social media their complaint about the medical team caring for them. All of these put us in a difficult spot, on top just trying to do a good job. How did David navigate this tension, to be excellent with a limited margin for error?

"There may be a calm surface, but the feet are moving fast below the surface. My being professionally anxious is in my patient's best interest. Patients are anxious in an unfocused, free-floating manner. I can use my concern for their well-being to assure I've been diligent in their care. In other words, harnessing my anxiety helps to focus my attention and avoid cursory thinking such as anchoring bias." He revels in it. He ups his game in response to the challenge. "That anxiety helps me to be mindful of all of what's going on with the patient, and to give them my full concentration, so that when I make a decision today, I am doing so considering all the information available. I've done my due diligence; I've dug into whatever needs to be dug into. But I'm also comfortable saying, *'I'm going to review you, and circumstances may change.'* Under many circumstances, being patient is rewarded." He was comfortable being uncomfortable.

He uses a familiar sport as an analogy to drive home the point. "In rugby, the oblong ball may bounce unpredictably when kicked or thrown. If you charge after a bouncing rugby ball, it may just as often bounce over your head as into your arms. If you wait for it to dissipate a bit of energy, instead of running toward it early in its journey, the bounces are less pronounced — giving you a better chance of catching it. In Medicine when the condition is not pressing, rushing to pin down a definitive diagnosis may lead to an incorrect diagnosis, an inappropriate course of action, and a waste of time and resources. On those occasions, if we were patient and gathered information that the passage of time and the evolution of disease provides, we can be more efficient."

"An example is when patients with fever are hospitalized and the radiologist provides a reading that '*Clinical correlation is needed as a pulmonary infection cannot be excluded*'. In the rush to provide a diagnosis and 'set' a plan of action, it is not uncommon for these patients to be categorised as having pneumonia — despite their lack of predisposition, symptoms, physical findings, or supportive laboratory results. It is convenient and effortless to hold onto that diagnosis, but it is only after they fail to respond or their syndrome evolves — often days later as it may be masked by the empiric pneumonia treatment — that it becomes even more apparent that pneumonia is not present. Patience, attention to detail, mindfulness, and a healthy dose of professional scepticism are invaluable skills."

One of the things doctors dislike doing for their patients is nothing. It feels as if we are doing a disservice to our patient by adopting *just* a 'wait and watch' approach whilst their body continues to be ravaged by an illness we have yet to fully work out. The mindset adopted by both the doctor and the patient becomes, metaphorically and physically, exhaustive — '*Surely, with our current advancements in medical care, we can get to the bottom of this?*' The approach taken becomes one of '*doing something is better than nothing*', thus inviting more diagnostic tests and therapeutic trials of medication for the patient. How does one overcome the element of guilt, that you've actually done your best for the patient, but are still unable to provide an answer?

"Humility." The response is simple.

"Humility is not defeatism or meekness." He clarifies further. "It is the recognition that at this time, the answer is not available. Doing things for the sake of looking busy is dealing with the physician's ego and sense of guilt, and not objectively addressing the situation in front of you."

David emphasises again. "Humility. Not fear, or *kiasu*-ism, or arrogance." He warned against such conceit — that Medicine has all the answers.

"As a doctor, one has to acknowledge that the practice of Medicine is rife with uncertainty, which if not managed, leads to fear and anxiety, sometimes resulting in irrational testing and unnecessary treatment. You have to embrace uncertainty and do the work required to address the situation at hand. Be open to continuous self-improvement, learning from each case regardless of the outcome, and have honest self-assessment of your weaknesses, all with the goal of excellence in mind."

We probe further by wondering if it was ever acceptable for a doctor to tell a patient that we do not know what is going on?

"I don't ever recall saying, '*I don't know*', full stop. A typical commentary is some form of, '*I'm not currently certain why you have the issue that you have, but I have a plan to sort this out. This process requires both of us to be patient. It also requires me to be persistent and to update you regularly, and for you to be observant of changes in your symptoms and to share those with me.*'"

He shares with us the importance of being honest with those under our care.

"It establishes realism — realistic time frames, expectations, and goals. Misleading patients results in loss of trust. When I discuss how we are going to resolve the uncertainty, they take the information well — thanking me for my forthrightness, recognition of their concerns, and reassurance that I am committed to seeing this through. People are grateful when you've given them your time and your consideration. They're so appreciative that you've given your attention to them and that you've actually heard them."

When did he come to this realisation, that uncertainty was something that he had to become comfortable with?

"I became comfortable with uncertainty probably during my last year of training in ID, or my first year as a young faculty person. Definitely when I moved to Singapore, because I was needing to make a lot of decisions with incomplete information without ready access to databases, and with the goal of doing what is in the patient's best interest. So, yeah, I became more comfortable with uncertainty then — by necessity."

Inevitably, mistakes are made because doctors are only human. Complaints from patients or their family members may or may not ensue as a result, but it could be a mentally challenging period for anyone, regardless. How did David, in the past, approach complaints made against him?

"Through self-reflection. I review if the concern is valid and if it is, then when, where, and why, I may have erred. I then attempt an objective assessment by asking peers if the problem was preventable. I then do a mental root-cause analysis, and work 'upstream' to put reasonable personal practice changes in place to prevent recurrences. In my experience, mistakes early in my career were less related to diagnosis and management, but more in not effectively communicating realistic expectations to the patient and family. I'm mindful of making an effort to communicate an accurate assessment of their loved one's condition and prognosis in a manner that does not remove hope but also does not give unsupportable expectations."

Has that approach changed now that he's a senior consultant?

"Yes. When I was a less experienced physician, I was not always able to see where and when potential problems might arise. Having been involved in a wide spectrum of medical and social situations at this stage of my career, these circumstances are more easily anticipated and prevented — usually via early, open and honest communication. Recognising the limitations of what Medicine, the profession, can and cannot do at a given point in time, is a good starting point."

How about when a complaint has been made against a junior member of his team? What is his *modus operandi*?

"First, I determine if the complaint has basis. If not, I speak with my team member and see how I can help them process the experience. If there is basis for the complaint, I have not found yelling, humiliation, or threats to be productive learning tools. These were used on me and my cohort during training. Likewise, brushing aside junior doctor errors is not helpful. I accept full responsibility for errors made on my watch — the buck stops with me." He claims to quote former US President Harry Truman here, who had a sign on his desk stating, '*The Buck Stops Here*', although the 46th President of the United States, Joseph Biden, lays claim to this quote as well. "It sends a powerful message to junior doctors when they know they are not treated as fodder. They will respond to corrective action accordingly."

The message he has for juniors who have made mistakes. "We work in teaching institutions, where junior doctors are learning via apprenticeships. We are human — mistakes will happen. Learn from the mistake, understand why it occurred, be mindful of what you are doing. Make efforts to ensure this is the last time you make this mistake."

One other aspect of clinical practice that we often struggle with was reconciling the differences that exist between what is described in textbooks in contrast to how patients present in real life. We turn, once again, towards the experience of Mikhail Bulgakov, who when attempting a life-saving tracheotomy in a little girl asphyxiating from diphtheria, and despite following textbook instructions, found instead that '*there was no windpipe anywhere to be seen. This wound of mine was quite unlike any illustration.*' By the same token, we are taught that AIDS-defining illnesses occur only when the immunity of a person with HIV has hit rock bottom — when he has AIDS. However, it is not inconceivable that in clinical practice, one may encounter a real-life patient with an AIDS-defining illness, such as Kaposi sarcoma or *Pneumocystis jirovecii* pneumonia, whose immune system, however, remains way above the threshold for getting such opportunistic infections. How do we move forward if we had no firm footing to begin with, where anything goes?

David's immediate reply dichotomizes the end-goals of learning. "All of what has been mentioned reflects a mindset which is useful for taking exams, but less helpful when managing patients." We had to be clear what the ultimate purpose of our learning is for — which was always to be for the benefit of our patients. He further elaborated.

"We have firm footing if we read, observe and reflect with an open mind. Textbooks describe classic presentations and often provide the probabilities of the typical individual signs, symptoms, laboratory findings and imaging being present. Texts are less able to give digestible insight into the wider spectra of symptoms, signs, laboratory and imaging combinations which we more often confront. Biologic systems are more complex than our technical writings often describe." In other words, patients do not always follow the textbook. "Medicine is a discipline of relativism, not absolutism. Returning to your example of AIDS — T-helper cell quantities are surrogates for net immunosuppression, but do not measure net immunosuppression holistically. Using CD4 lymphocyte levels for anything other than as surrogates in the scenario described would not acknowledge the assay's limitations."

"Our need to communicate to others how to recognise disease requires reductionism to be effective. Reductionism provides a common language for us but it is only a starting point. The purpose of a medical apprenticeship is to learn the language and basic concepts, then one must immerse oneself to see, appreciate, and recognise, the gamut of possible presentations. The professional makes that leap from the concrete 'must' to the more abstract 'possible'; a technician does not."

We move on to a topic that straddles across the many generations of doctors, affecting both modern professionals of the art and keepers of the ancient practice of Medicine. The young protagonist in the '*A Country Doctor's Notebook*' laments, '*Kerosene lamps may be very cosy, but I prefer electricity.*' Indeed, we similarly have to navigate the tension between being comfortable with what has been traditionally practised, tried and tested, compared with new knowledge and technology. How should one go about it?

For this, David says with candour, "If you want to stick with what you always do, I urge you to gain experience with other effective strategies. You only learn their pros and cons by employing and observing. Our activities are increasingly evidence-based or at least evidence-influenced. Nostalgia has no place in our work except to entertain our trainees, as well as to remind us: that out-of-the-box diagnostic and management options which are no longer in common use can at least be considered when circumstances dictate."

Many a times, a trainee is entirely fixated upon institutional algorithms or eminence-based medicine (relying on the experiences of a senior doctor, rather than the latest evidence in the medical literature). What were some of the ways that we could overcome suboptimal or outdated institutional practices?

"It is important for trainees to be aware there is often more than one approach to diagnosing and managing patients while remaining true to ID fundamental concepts. However, the discussions regarding or their experience employing these approaches may be limited due to the vagaries of institutional practice. Institutional practice can become monolithic for many reasons: economic; resource availability; ease of auditing guideline adherence; lack of experience with different approaches; expert opinion — with attendant contextual bias — in the absence of quality evidence, et cetera. Having faculty with exposure to practices outside of their mother institution and from mentors who look beyond standard operating procedure will provide perspectives which enhance patient care, departmental discussions, and the trainee experience."

We potentially open a can of worms here with our follow-up question. What if a consultant is doing something wrong but refuses to acknowledge it? What could and should a junior doctor do, being in a position of vulnerability?

"Speak with the Programme Director or the Head of Department, if you think someone is causing harm to patients, and they're not responding to or are defensive of polite inquiries. You will be helping patients, the department, the hospital and the community." Ultimately, this hinges upon the other medical ethical principles of *beneficence* and *non-maleficence*. Performing a deed that benefits the patient, whilst refraining from doing harm. He reinforces our professional obligations, which is our duty of care to the patient. "As a trainee, you do have an obligation to patients, and if you see something happening, you do need to do something about it."

David shares with us some of the issues on his side of the fence. "Sadly, being an old White guy with a long Singapore Infectious Diseases history may result in younger trainees hesitating in questioning me...though I hope not. And I make a point when working with someone whom I've not worked with before to ask me to clarify if they are not absolutely certain and comfortable, based on our discussion, with what we are doing."

This is what he perceives to be his '*White Man's Burden*'. His solution to breaking down the barriers of formality? "I try my best to engage and remind the team, '*Look, we're all earnestly working to give the patient their best outcome. We are making decisions with incomplete information. My job is to assure we do so as safely, expeditiously and resource efficiently as we can. There is often more than one way to achieve these goals — let's talk objectively about them.*' By doing so, we expand the trainee's horizons, allow the experience to be more intellectually engaging and hopefully provide the patient more personalized care. Ultimately, I'm going to prison when something goes wrong." Laughter, with an ounce of truth.

"What I'm trying to do is to get trainees to commit to a course of action, tell me what their other diagnostic and therapeutic management options are, and to defend their decisions. If they are able to address my challenges to their plan to my satisfaction, then we implement their plan. Having to explain and defend their approach requires greater insight. Ownership under a watchful eye provides confidence. For educational purposes, I prefer not to dictate care unless the trainee is not ready to assume that role and defend their choices."

Our discussion now brings us to a phenomenon that is currently gaining traction in our times. It is not a novelty, but has acquired a novel name — 'quiet quitting'. In a push back against the professional demands of Medicine as a calling, some doctors have begun to view Medicine as nothing more than a job. The boundaries between work and personal well-being are firmly drawn, with the time afforded for the former not allowed to seep into the latter. This may manifest as the resident who declines to see a patient referral made to his specialty the second it is passed office hours, or the resident who consciously refuses to engage in the non-patient-related aspects of work, such as the education of medical students or junior residents. In other words, it is a refusal to go above and beyond at work, a form of resistance to work conditions that increasingly encroach on people's lives. We put forth this question to David outrightly — is 'quiet quitting' tolerable for him?

"No."

He jettisons this behaviour outright. This was another concept that was quite foreign to him. He gives his rationale for his rejection.

"Institutional medicine works best for all when we take responsibility for the tasks assigned us. The Singapore Medical Council's Physician's Pledge which is required to qualify for medical practitioner registration includes at least two components which appear to address the mindset you reference, *'make the health of my patient my first consideration'*, and *'respect my colleagues as my professional brothers and sisters'*. Therefore, the resident would not be in compliance with the Pledge. Steps should be taken to facilitate them achieving compliance."

His reply comes across as rather doctrinaire thinking, but we are with him on this. Without sounding too patronizing, we quote *'Atomic Habits'*[5] by James Clear here — *'stepping up when it's annoying or painful or draining to do so, that's what makes the difference between a professional and an amateur.*' There is a certain level of necessary discomfort that is required of you when you sign up to be a doctor, be it something as straight-forward as handling blood or excrements (with gloves of course), or working past duty hours for the sake of the patient who has turned ill at the end of the shift.

But still we push back. Some doctors feel like a cog in the wheel whose job is to meet very high productivity standards, ensuring goals of efficiency, such as waiting times for clinic visits or shortening hospital stays, are met at the cost of the doctor-patient relationship. This places a lot of pressure on the residents and in order to protect them, and over here we cite some local examples, departments may put in place certain limits. This may be in the form of restricting the number of new outpatient visits for residents to see per session, or limiting the number of new specialty referrals a resident sees in a day. Any 'excess' workload then gets taken up by a peer or a senior. Some residents take this demarcation very seriously and follow it to the letter. But it may also be construed as a form of 'quiet quitting'. An additional downside of this is that the resident's learning opportunity becomes curtailed. Where do we draw the line?

"There has always been disagreement as to what constitutes educational activity, and when does the work become non-educational service work in return for the education provided, and when does it become abusive. Each party in that arrangement has a different perspective on the proper balance. The line is drawn where the parties explicitly or tacitly agree it to be drawn. I don't believe the working environment in which I was trained in is comparable to those training in the 2020s; therefore, I cannot in good conscience use the number of referrals as the standard."

He jests at this point.

"We need to develop an ID resident education/work-product/abuse matrix."

We laugh. But in all seriousness, what would his approach to the 'quiet quitter' be?

"An individual's circumstances, or their vision of their life's work, may change as they age. In general, I would bring this to the attention of their Programme Director, and a one-on-one conversation would take place between the Programme Director and resident to determine if there was a misunderstanding of what took place, or of expectations, or if their 'quiet quitting' was due to 'other reasons' such as external pressures or well-being. If due to a misunderstanding of expectations, then the clarification and the restatement of expectations should occur with the resident's explicit acknowledgement. If there was not a misunderstanding, and the behaviour is due to 'other reasons', then reasonable accommodations should be offered as able. If there was not a misunderstanding, and the behaviour was not due to 'other reasons', the conversation should then delve into whether the programme's and the trainee's goals align."

An even darker incarnation of 'quiet quitting' faced by doctors is that of apathy. In the novel '*Heart of Darkness*'[6], Joseph Conrad writes, '*Even extreme grief may ultimately vent itself in violence, but more often it takes the form of apathy.*' Mikhail Bulgakov in '*A Country Doctor's Notebook*', reflecting on his tumultuous year at the countryside hospital practicing as its only medical doctor, comments almost nonchalantly, after finding out that a patient had died at the hands of another colleague, '*No doctor murders anyone, and if someone dies on you, then it's just bad luck.*' Young doctors face a heavy workload, and coupled with sleep deprivation and disillusionment with their work, may start to burn out. This then manifests as apathy, with a display of indifference towards our colleagues and our patients. We stop caring. We lose our original drive and motivation. What could we do if we start losing the capacity to care?

There is a long pause here. It was an issue close to the heart of many doctors, and, dare we say it, something that he had possibly encountered and had to overcome himself.

He commiserates. "I know the feeling, and it's painful. There are many reasons for burnout. These should be explored — either with self-reflection, or with someone trained to help. Once the causes of burnout are identified, and if amenable to intervention — such as addressing life-work balance, moral injury, lack of self-care, et cetera — then efforts can be made to remedy."

"I would say that I believe we're in an atmosphere now that we are able to speak with our Programme Directors and say, '*I'm having trouble. I'm worried about my physical well-being. I'm worried about my mental well-being. And I need help.'* As much as we don't want to widely broadcast it, there are opportunities for others to do the work, to carry the burden, to lighten the load a bit for our colleagues who are suffering. It may be uncomfortable but that's why they're hired. To be able to step up. We do that for each other as we would want them to do for us should the circumstance arise."

Reassuringly, from the vantage point of a consultant, the situation is viewed differently. "I know the Programme Directors recognise that trainees may need help from time to time and are prompt in their efforts to provide the help needed. Unfortunately, there is still a stigma which delays acknowledgement and steps to address the situation — it's not helpful. Early recognition and intervention are to everyone's benefit."

Even consultants are not spared such tribulations.

"I'd mentioned before, one of the things I had problems with in '94 [when he first left Singapore], was that I couldn't say no. Pretty soon, the commitments add up. It was more than a little tiresome. So, you just have to figure out a constructive way to tap the brakes."

How do or should senior doctors handle such a situation?

"Generally, we will recognise symptoms of burnout in ourselves; however, if we have a lack of self-awareness or are in denial, then it is possible not to perceive it. If we feel professional norms expect us to 'work through it' or are fearful of stigma, then acknowledgement and addressing the causative activity will be delayed. In those scenarios, the decline in the quality of work and or in the interactions we have with family, co-workers and patients will ring alarm bells that it is more than just 'stress' or fatigue." He stresses again the importance of naming the issue. "The best first step is acknowledgement."

How had he managed to guard against apathy setting in all these years?

"Realise each day what an exceptional life society allows us to lead as doctors. Listen to your friends in business, finance, law, engineering, et cetera, talk about their work. I think the world of my friends not in Medicine, but I find their work less intellectually stimulating over the long haul. I'm sure it satisfies them and I am grateful that they do it, but having their jobs would not get me out of bed in the morning. As doctors, we witness and participate during intimate, vulnerable times in our patients' lives. Times of birth, death, acceptance of mortality…We are often able to return them from poor health to wellness. We are generally held in high regard by society, compensated well, work in a safe environment, and are provided an opportunity to constantly learn. My advice to avoid career apathy — step back, open your eyes, weigh your alternative options and appreciate what an extraordinary privilege we are granted. If other opportunities excite you, by all means pursue them."

In '*A Country Doctor's Notebook*', Mikhail Bulgakov states, upon arrival at his new assignment at the countryside hospital, '*Man's basic needs are few. The first of them is fire…Besides fire, man also needs to find his bearings.*' On superficial reading, he meant the literal need for a flame to keep warm, and an understanding of his surroundings so as to navigate his way around. Yet, on closer inspection, he meant more than that. He realised that, in order to survive and to thrive, he needed to keep alive the spark — the passion — that had brought him to be a doctor in the first place. And the only way to keep the flame burning was to keep his eye on the prize, that is, to be of service to his patients.

This was the message David was trying to get across.

Notes

[1] M. Bulgakov. (2013) 'A Country Doctor's Notebook'. Melville House Pub.

[2] Interview with Dr Edmund Monteiro [13 Apr 2024]

[3] Interview with Ms Iris Verghese [8 May 2024]

[4] T. Kidder. (2011) 'Mountains Beyond Mountains'. Profile Books.

[5] J. Clear. (2018) 'Atomic Habits'. Penguin Random House.

[6] J. Conrad. (1995) 'Heart of Darkness'. Wordsworth Editions.

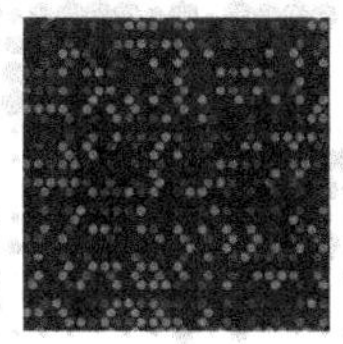

EPILOGUE

–

vincit qui se vincit
'he conquers who conquers himself'

The afternoon's dialogue draws to a close, and '*Barbie*', the movie, beckons, for David. On hindsight, it seemed like the appropriate choice, after an afternoon of splitting atoms and firing neurons. '*Oppenheimer*' would have been too onerous for the remaining functional grey matter. Furthermore, the slogan for the original Barbie doll reads, '*You can be anything.*' It was right on cue with the theme of the afternoon. David had left us lots of food for thought, and many pieces of gum to chew on. But there was always plenty of room for dessert. As much as he had allowed, we had uncovered lots about the founding father of Infectious Diseases in Singapore, but yet, David still remained quite a bit of an enigma. Perhaps the old, White guy persona was true after all – the differences between the generations, and the divide between the Oriental and the Occidental, was a gap too far to bridge. Nevertheless, he had allowed us to make inroads, to pick his brains, and then bequeathed us his inheritance of wisdom.

A fact not widely publicised about the Infectious Diseases specialty is the propensity for many, if not all, of its practitioners to treat it like a bit of trophy hunting. There was a world of pathogens out there waiting to be 'collected', some were a dime a dozen, while others were like the proverbial unicorn that was hunted for every time we heard hoofbeats. It was all for a bit of fun. But, along those lines, we drew some inference for our next inquiry.

Are there any pathogens that has still eluded you, that still motivates you to come to work every morning?

"I hate to say it but, at a certain point in time, host-pathogen interactions have a certain repetitiveness. There may be a different constellation of outcomes, a little more of this, a little less of that. But I don't know that I haven't seen every organ system infected with virus, bacteria, mycobacteria, or fungi. No, there's not a lot I haven't seen, and there're certain ones I've seen enough of already."

Dare we say it, but was David actually getting bored of Infectious Diseases?

"But I'm still learning every day. Some in infectious diseases, but also population health issues, and how government works, how decisions are made, how policy is made. That is what motivates me, trying to understand all the different moving parts and how they're weighted, because no one states it explicitly. It's not written anywhere. You must figure it out — *'How did we get to this point? And should we change? And if we change, how will we get to the next point?'* So that part engages me."

Perhaps he had taken a leaf out of Dr William Osler's notebook — "*The young doctor should look about early for an avocation, a pastime, that will take him away from patients, pills, and potions.*" David's own mosaic of knowledge and experiences were still unfinished, and instead of fighting against one bug for one patient at a time, he was more motivated now to engage his mortal enemies on a grander scale. It was not a pastime, but it was a guard for him against apathy.

What has been the most rewarding aspect of the work for you?

"Patient care — all aspects of that. Being in a position to help people, whether it's returning them to full health, making them less miserable, accompanying them on their final journey, or just reassuring them. Teaching has been one of the most rewarding aspects of my work. I very much enjoy how we all learn differently. I can't, for instance, go and sit in at a lecture and gain much from it. It's often a waste of time for me. Whereas if I read something, I can absorb it quickly. We all acquire information differently, and the way we organise information fascinates me. One of the parts I enjoy most about teaching is quickly trying to determine the most efficient manner in which to transmit information to individual trainees. Being willing to step away from your own process of assimilating information and pitch it in a way that may allow another person to gain insight. Hearing people say, '*Ah, that makes sense.*' That part is fun."

The moral lesson, '养不教，父之过' [yǎng bù jiào, fù zhī guò], from the classic Chinese text, '三字经' [sān zì jīng], '*Three Character Classic*', written in the 13th century, springs to mind. '*It is the father's fault if he only raises his children without cultivating them*'. This would resonate with David.

What is the one important piece of advice that you have for future generations?

"*Throughout your career, in the management of your patients, it is always important to remain uncomfortable.*"

It was his age-old adage, something he never failed to remind those under his tutelage. Something that he has reminded us throughout this whole interview, whether through his advice, or through his actions.

"It is a fundamental truth. We are privileged to be involved at a vulnerable point in another human's life. And we should not be so certain that we no longer think about them and their condition. We should always question our diagnosis and management. If nothing more, to say, '*I have done my due diligence. I have done what is right for this patient. As a professional, I've carried out my duties.*' If nothing more, just to say, '*Okay, I'm happy with how things are going today.*' But tomorrow, or whenever I see them next, I'll think about it again and revisit it. I think it's important to be always uncomfortable. I don't mean 'uncomfortable', '*Oh gosh, I can't sleep*', but I mean being 'uncomfortable' is to give them the courtesy of your attention and be earnest about it."

This has been something that you've always been telling us, and is now something that we've gone on to tell others as well.

"The memory of one in the minds of others or in the cultural sphere is the only empirically established path to immortality."

Be uncomfortable.

Be all you can be.

You're a better person because of it.

"I'm not interested in adulation. I'm proud that I was here, and that I worked hard to make things better than when I first arrived. That what I contributed has made a difference."

Relevance.

And that's how this all came about.

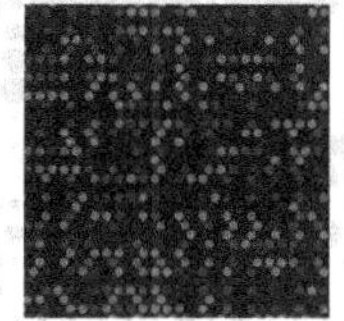

ACKNOWLEDGEMENTS

We embarked on this project on the basis of a whim, and have been met with nothing but overwhelming support and encouragement. This project has led us to encounter many important figures who have been modest about their enormous contributions to our specialty — we are grateful that they have shared their invaluable time and their stories about our Singapore Infectious Diseases history, and of David. In particular, Prof Brenda Ang, Prof Chee Yam Cheng, Prof Chong Chia Yin, Prof Hsu Li Yang, Prof Koh Liang Piu, Dr Lam Mun San, Prof Leo Yee-Sin, Prof Raymond Lin, Dr Shirley Yeo Llizo, Dr Edmund Monteiro, Prof Helen Oh, Ms Iris Verghese, Dr Wong Sin Yew, and Prof John Wong. We are additionally grateful as well to Prof Paul Tambyah for graciously writing the foreword for this book, sharing his many golden insights and pearls of wisdom, and in general, always being a staunch supporter in almost anything we do.

Special thanks to the Society of Infectious Disease (Singapore) for allowing us access to the SIDS archives, as well as sponsoring the project. We are grateful too for the support of the ID division at NUH.

We are especially grateful to Ms Angela Sng, the niece of Dr Edmund Monteiro, for linking us up with her uncle, as well as to Ms Larissa Breedlove, Communications Manager of the Department of Medicine at

Weill Cornell Medicine, for helping us obtain photos of David during his time in Cornell.

A shout out to our peers who have been wonderful sounding boards. These would include: Dr Alicia Ang, Dr Chan Yu Kit, Dr Chew Ka Lip, Dr Chia Po Ying, Dr Choy Chiaw Yee, Dr Priscillia Lye, Dr Deborah Ng, Dr Stephanie Sutjipto, Dr Glorijoy Tan and Dr Tay Jun Yang. To Dr Matthew Koh, thank you for taking on the arduous task of being the final bastion of proof-reading for this book. To Dr Goh Yihui, thanks for sharing with us your multifaceted talents, and for being the ultimate David Allen fan and stalwart supporter in this project.

Thanks also to our family, especially Nic's wife, Sarah, and son, Jeremy; and Gab's wife, Chun Yi, and children, Nathan, Daniel and Elizabeth. Hope you get to understand a little more about what bugs your husband/father after reading this.

As the Chinese proverb goes — '听君一席话，胜读十年书' [tīng jūn yī xí huà, shèng dú shí nián shū] *Listening to the words of a wise person is superior to ten years of studying*. We have definitely gained more than a decade's worth of insight from these interview sessions with David. We have said much, but will state again that we have been extremely privileged to have been the recipients of his patience and generosity.

Finally, any errors or misrepresentations within the pages of this book are entirely the fault of the authors and the authors alone.

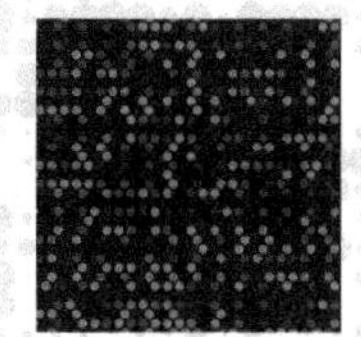

PHOTOGRAPHS

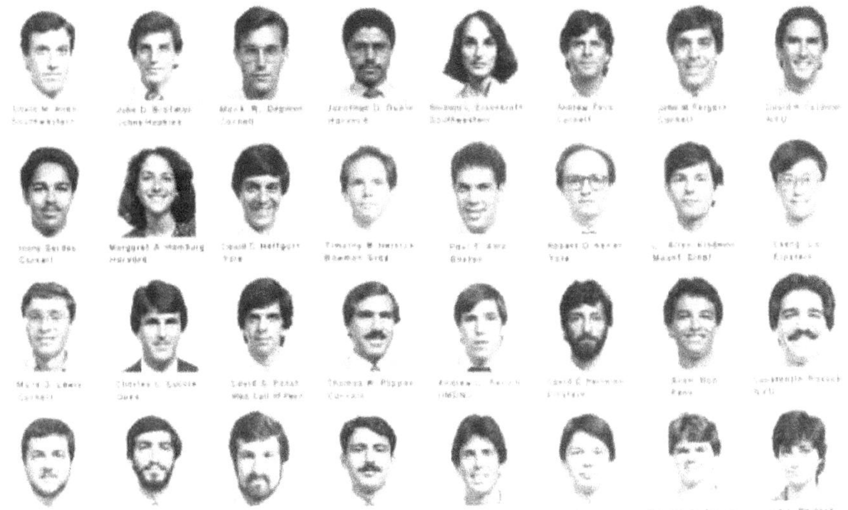

New York Hospital-Cornell Medical Center First Year Assistant Physicians on the Medical House Staff, 1984–1985. Prof David Allen's portrait is at the top left-hand corner. [Courtesy of Ms Larissa Breedlove and the Medical Center Archives of NewYork-Presbyterian/Weill Cornell]

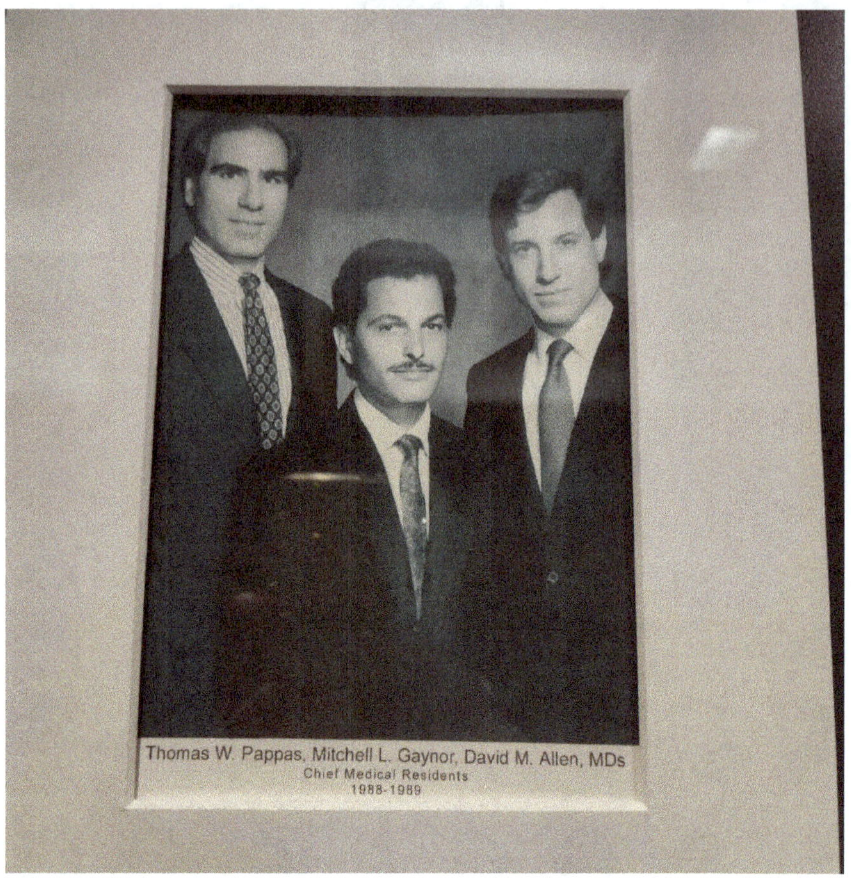

Prof David Allen, far right, and his fellow Chief Medical Residents, 1988–1989, adorn the wall of the Chair's Office in the Weill Department of Medicine at NewYork-Presbyterian/Weill Cornell Medical Center. The photo of Prof Allen's cohort sits among more than two dozen photos of chief residents and Department chairs dating back to the 1950s. [Courtesy of Ms Larissa Breedlove]

NO. 5.00pm
DATE 12.1.90

Members Present at the Inaugural Meeting

Name	Address	Telephone # (H)/(O)
D. LEO YEE SIN	CDC / TTSH .	Pg 2030495
Dr. LAM MUN SAN	MU4 TTSH	Pg. 6040575
Dr. Sng Ewe Hui	Pathology Dept.	3214900
DR WONG SIN YEW	MU 3 SGH	3214700 6913
TAN AI LING	Pathology	3214908
LING AI EE	Pathology / Virology	3214940/1
DR. S. DORAISINGHAM	Pathology / Virology	3214940
DR LING MOI LIN	PATHOLOGY / BACTERIOLOGY	3214953
CHAN KWAI PENG	PATHOLOGY / BACTERIOLOGY	3214945 0819
DR. M. NADARAJAH	Pathology / Serology	3214921
DR RAYMOND LIN TZER PIN	PATHOLOGY / BACTERIOLOGY	3214945
DR EDMUND H. MONTEIRO	CDC / TTSH	3508430
David M. Allen	CDC / TTSH	IS PAGT 2008911
CHEE YAM CHENG	TAN TOCK SENG HOSPITAL	2566011
Howe Hwee Kien	Tan Tock Seng Hospital	2566011
Chng Hiok Hee	Tan Tock Seng Hosp	2566011
Feng Pao Hsii	Tan Tock Seng Hosp.	2566011

Attendance of the Inaugural Society of Infectious Diseases (Singapore) Meeting (12th January 1990) [Courtesy of SIDS]

SINGAPORE SOCIETY OF INFECTIOUS DISEASE
c/o Department of Medicine IV
Tan Tock Seng Hospital
Moulmein Road, Singapore 1130

Minutes of the Inaugural Meeting

The inaugural meeting of the society was held on 12th January 1990 at 4.30 pm at Conference Room, Staff Recreation Centre, Tan Tock Seng Hospital. The meeting was chaired by Prof Feng Pao Hsii.

Members present :   Dr Leo Yee Sin
Dr Sng Ewe Hui
Dr Ling Ai Ee
Dr Ling Moi Lin
Dr M Nadarajah
Dr Edmund H Monteiro
Dr Chee Yam Cheng
Dr Chng Hiok Hee
Dr Lam Mun San
Dr Tan Ai Ling
Dr S Doraisingham
Dr Chan Kwai Peng
Dr Raymond Lin Tzer Pin
Dr David M Allen
Dr Howe Hwee Siew
Dr Wong Sin Yew
Dr Thirumoorthy
Prof Feng Pao Hsii

1.   Prof Feng Pao Hsii opened the meeting by tracing the development of the interest in infectious diseases in Singapore. Currently there is sustained momentum in the development of this discipline locally and he felt it is timely to have the Singapore Society of Infectious Disease formed to maintain this interest.

2.   Prof Feng explained the necessary steps and requirements in establishing a new society :-

(1)   Inaugural meeting

(2)   Setting up a Protem Committee

(3)   Drafting of Constitution of the society

(4)   Application to the Registrar of Societies for approval

Minutes of the Inaugural Society of Infectious Diseases (Singapore) Meeting (12th January 1990) [Courtesy of SIDS]

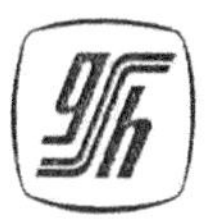 Singapore General Hospital

16 January 1993

Stuart Levin, M.D.
Program Director, Internal Medicine Residency Program
Rush-Presbyterian-St. Luke's Medical Center
1653 W. Congress Pkwy
Chicago, Illinois 60612

Dear Dr. Levin:

I am writing in support of Dr. Paul Ananth Tambyah's application for a residency position in your Internal Medicine program. I have known Dr. Tambyah for two years.

My comments are based upon my experience within New York Hospital/Cornell University Medical Center as Assistant Professor of Medicine, Chief Medical Resident, Infectious Diseases Fellow, Medical Resident and member of the Residency Selection Committee under Dr. R. Gordon Douglas, Jr. from 1983-89.

Dr. Tambyah graduated from medical school in 1988. Since graduation he has completed his housemanship (internship equivalent), served an obigatory two years as medical officer in the Singapore Armed Forces and has most recently been a medical officer in Internal Medicine within the National University Hospital (Singapore) training program. As a trainee in internal medicine, he has rotated onto a variety of medical subspeciality services in addition to general medicine. Dr. Tambyah has completed the first portion of the requisite two exams to be eligible for membership in the Royal College of Physicians (MRCP-UK) and has a ECFMG certificate. His current status is equivalent to a mature 2nd year resident in the U.S. training system.

The Singapore training program is fashioned after the British system. Training in internal medicine is comprehensive. The spectrum of disease seen in Singapore and the responsibility assumed by a Singapore medical trainee are similar to a tertiary referral hospital in the United States. A local internist who successfully completes the rigorous examination gauntlet is comparable to a top 5% medical resident in the United States.

In the above setting Dr. Tambyah has distinguished himself as an excellent physician. He has a solid command of general internal medicine and is an enthusiastic teacher of medical students. His interest in internal medicine is further exemplified by his involvement in clinical projects, some of which have led to publication. In line with current trends in American medicine, his approach to patient care is pragmatic and cost-effective.

Singapore General Hospital Pte Ltd
Outram Road Singapore 0316. Tel: 2223322
Telex: RS 28847 GENHOS Fax: 2221720

A Tradition of Caring & Excellence

Dr. Stuart Levin
Page 2

Dr. Tambyah's life has not been one-dimensional. He has participated in international debate competitions and has been recognized for his public service efforts. Although English is his first language, he is also conversant in various Chinese dialects.

While Paul is receiving excellent training in internal medicine in Singapore, the local approach to problem solving is different from that utilized in the U.S. The analytical and literature-based approach employed in most U.S. training programs provides a perspective that would be a useful supplement to local teaching tactics. Paul wishes to pursue a career in Infectious Diseases. This area is currently understaffed in Singapore.

Exposure to basic scientists, clinical investigators and thought-provoking clinicians will allow Dr. Tambyah to prepare for his role as a teacher/investigator in internal medicine and infectious diseases. Dr. Tambyah is a well-rounded applicant of the highest caliber who will bring experience, discipline, maturity and enthusiasm to an internal medicine residency program. He will easily compare with top candidates from the U.S. for residency positions. I recommend him without reservation.

Sincerely yours,

David M. Allen, M.D., Mem ACP
Dipl. ABIM (Int. Med., Inf. Dis.)
Consultant Physician
Singapore General Hospital

Head, Dept of Infectious Diseases
Communicable Disease Centre

Assistant Prof of Medicine (Adj.)
Cornell University Medical Center

Dr. Levin,
Hope all is well. I believe this young man would be a real asset to Singapore in the long run. He's more engaging than most Singaporean' medical trainees. I think he would work well in a residency and (eventually) fellowship. Best wishes for the New Year
Warm Regards,
David

Letter of Recommendation written by Prof David Allen for Prof Paul Tambyah for his application for Infectious Diseases training in the United States (16th January 1993)
[Courtesy of Prof Paul Tambyah]

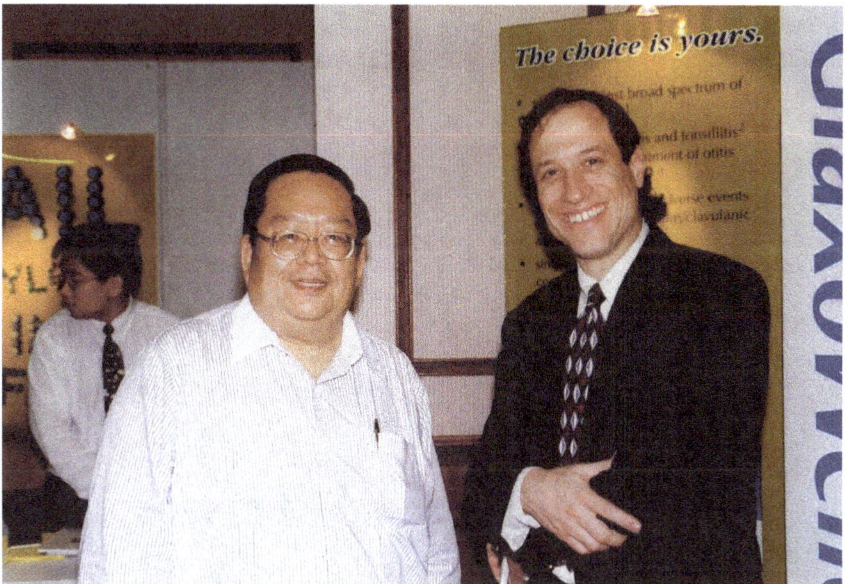

Prof David Allen with Prof Feng Pao Hsii at the opening ceremony of Practice Update in Infectious Disease, 1998 [Courtesy of SIDS]

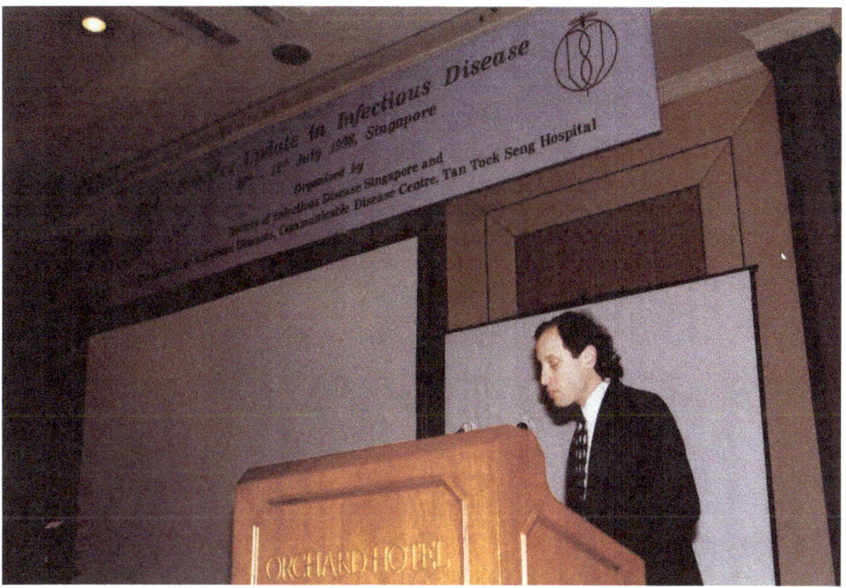

Speaker at the Practice Update in Infectious Disease, 1998 [Courtesy of SIDS]

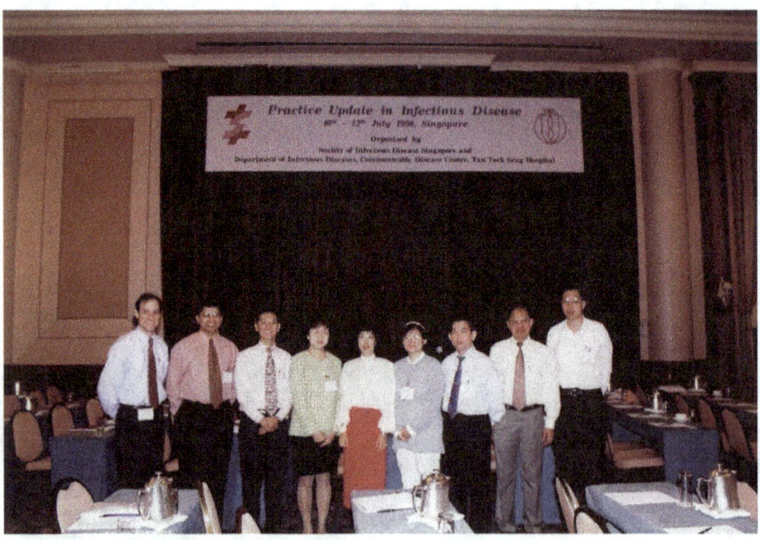

Practice Update in Infectious Disease, 1998 [Courtesy of SIDS]
From left to right: Prof David Allen, Dr Asok Kurup, Dr Wong Sin Yew, Dr Lam Mun San, Prof Brenda Ang, Prof Leo Yee-Sin, Dr Lee Cheng Chuan, Dr Edmund Monteiro, Dr Teoh Yee Leong (Ministry of Environment)

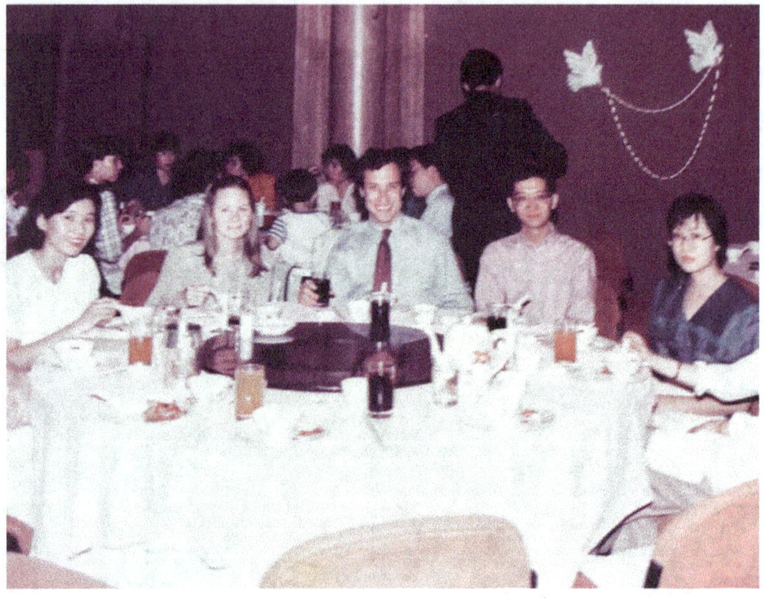

Dinner function [Courtesy of Prof David Allen]
From left to right: Dr Lau Yung Sang, Ms J.C. Puckett (Prof David Allen's wife), Prof David Allen, Dr Wong Sin Yew, and Dr Lam Mun San

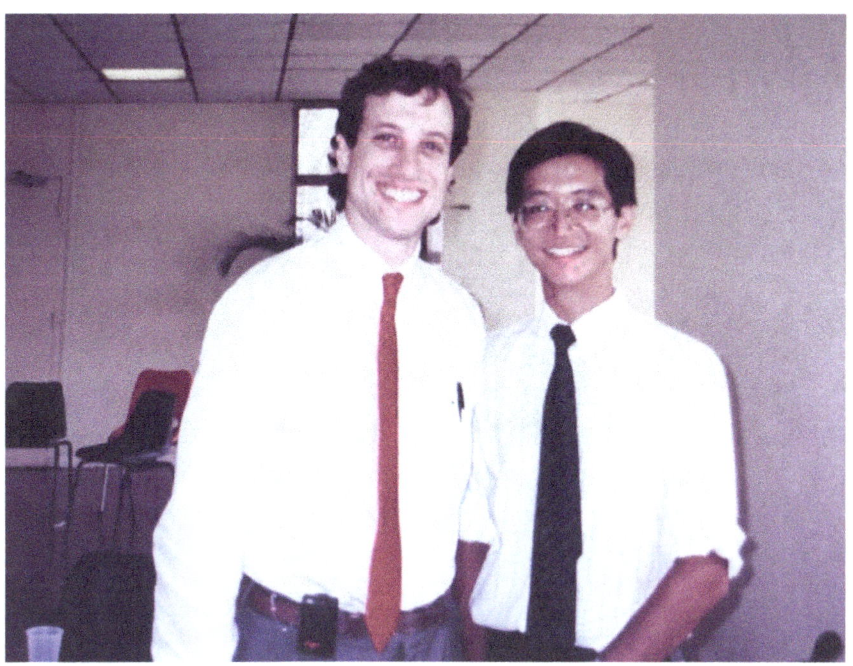

Prof David Allen and Dr Wong Sin Yew [Courtesy of Prof David Allen]

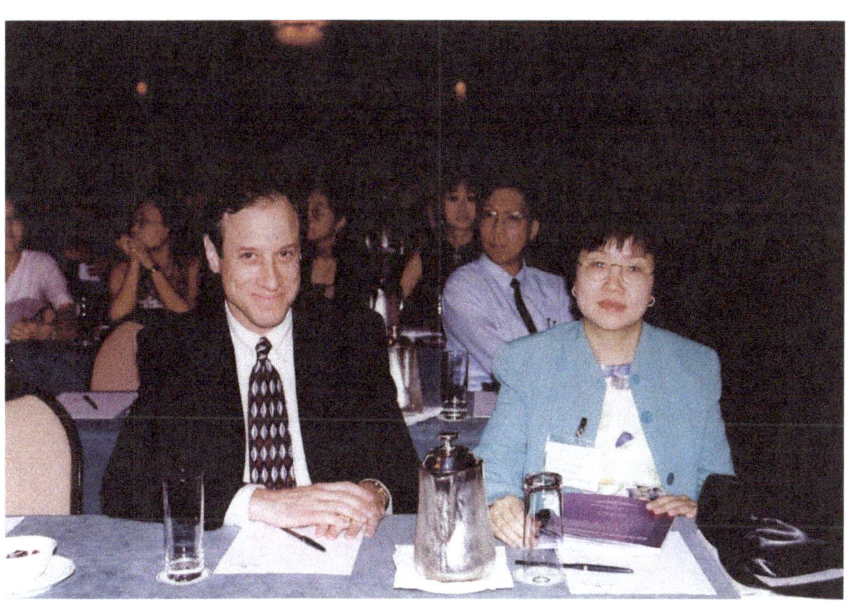

Prof David Allen and Dr Lam Mun San [Courtesy of SIDS]

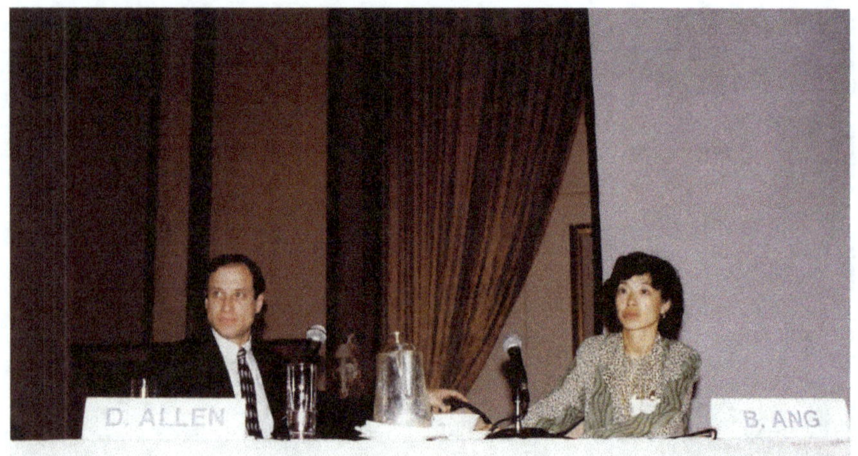

Prof David Allen and Prof Brenda Ang [Courtesy of SIDS]

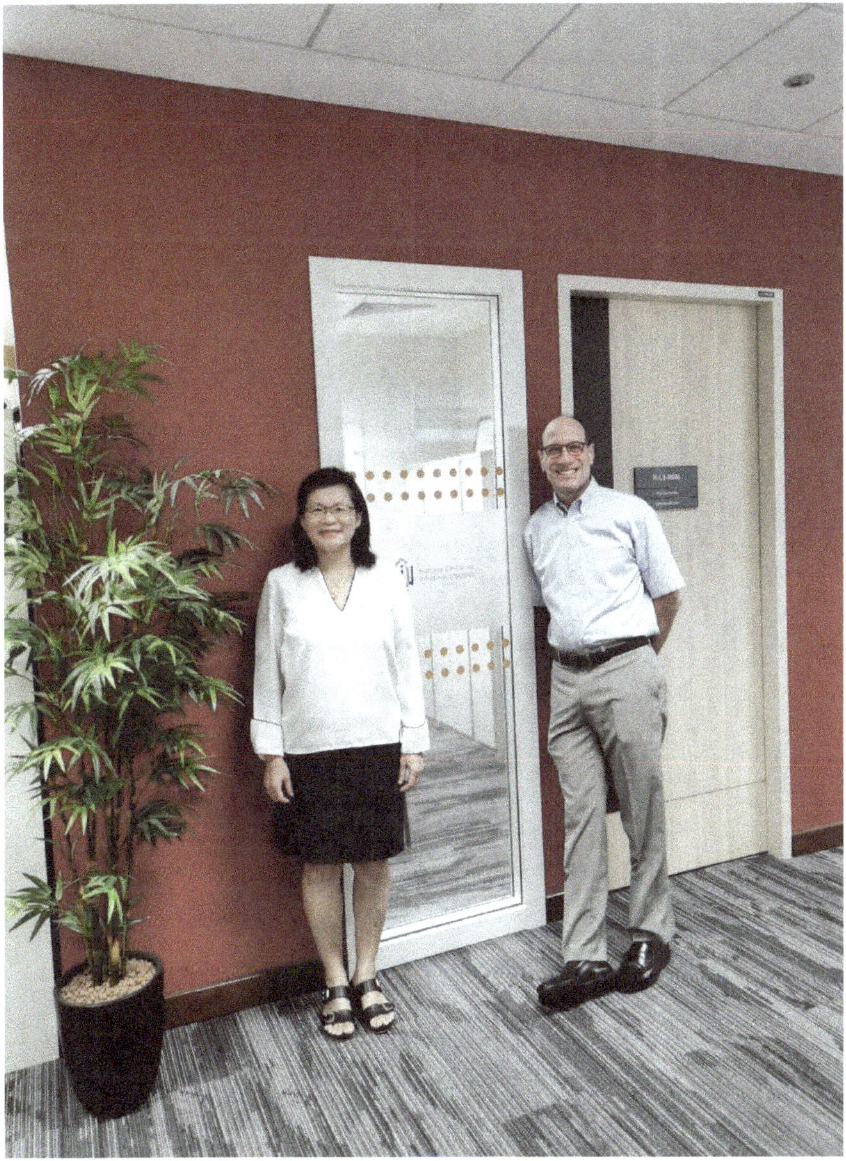

Prof Leo Yee-Sin and Prof David Allen [Courtesy of National Centre for Infectious Diseases]

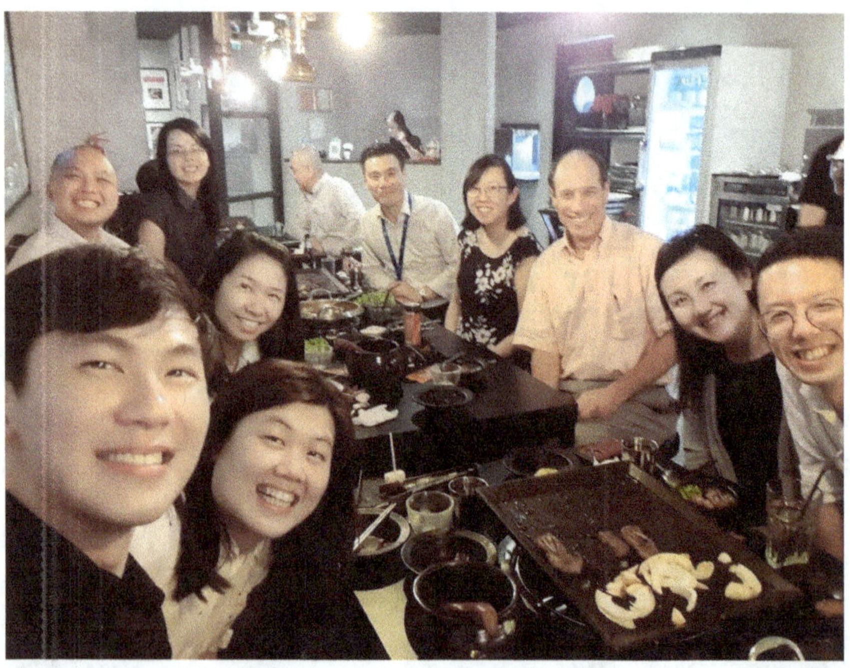

With the NCID ID Community [Courtesy of Prof David Allen]
Clockwise from far left (looking at the camera): Dr Tay Jun Yang, Dr Lee Pei Hua, Ms Vivien Heng, Dr Wong Chen Seong, Dr Monica Chan, Dr Lee Tau Hong, Dr Chan Yu Kit, Prof David Allen, Dr Stephanie Sutjipto, Dr Sean Ong

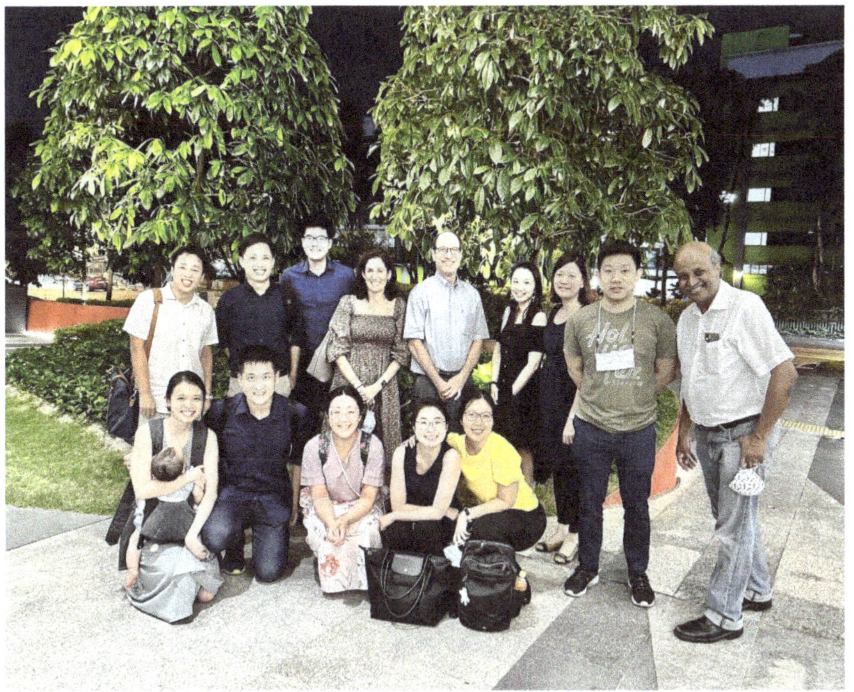

With the NUH ID Community [Courtesy of Prof Sophia Archuleta]

Back row from left to right: Dr Lionel Lum, Dr Nicholas Ngiam, Dr Gabriel Yan, Prof Sophia Archuleta, Prof David Allen, Dr Jolene Oon, Dr Catherine Ong, Dr Nares Smitasin, Prof Paul Tambyah

Front row from left to right: Dr Tan Jia Neng and child, Dr Tham Sai Meng, Dr Alicia Ang, Dr Priscillia Lye, Ms Joy Yong

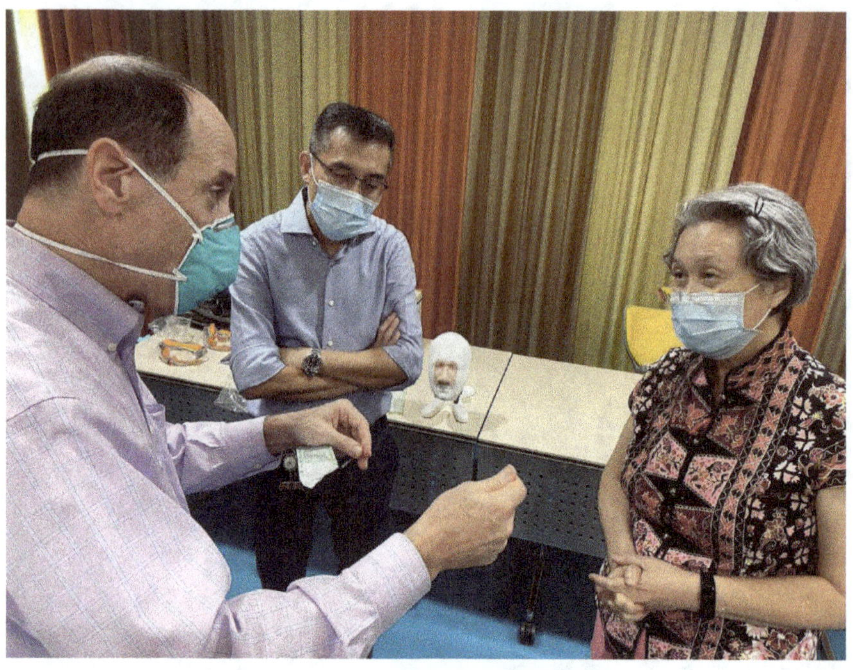

Prof David Allen explaining about COVID-19 testing with locally made 3D-printed nasal swabs to Mdm Ho Ching [Courtesy of Prof John Wong]

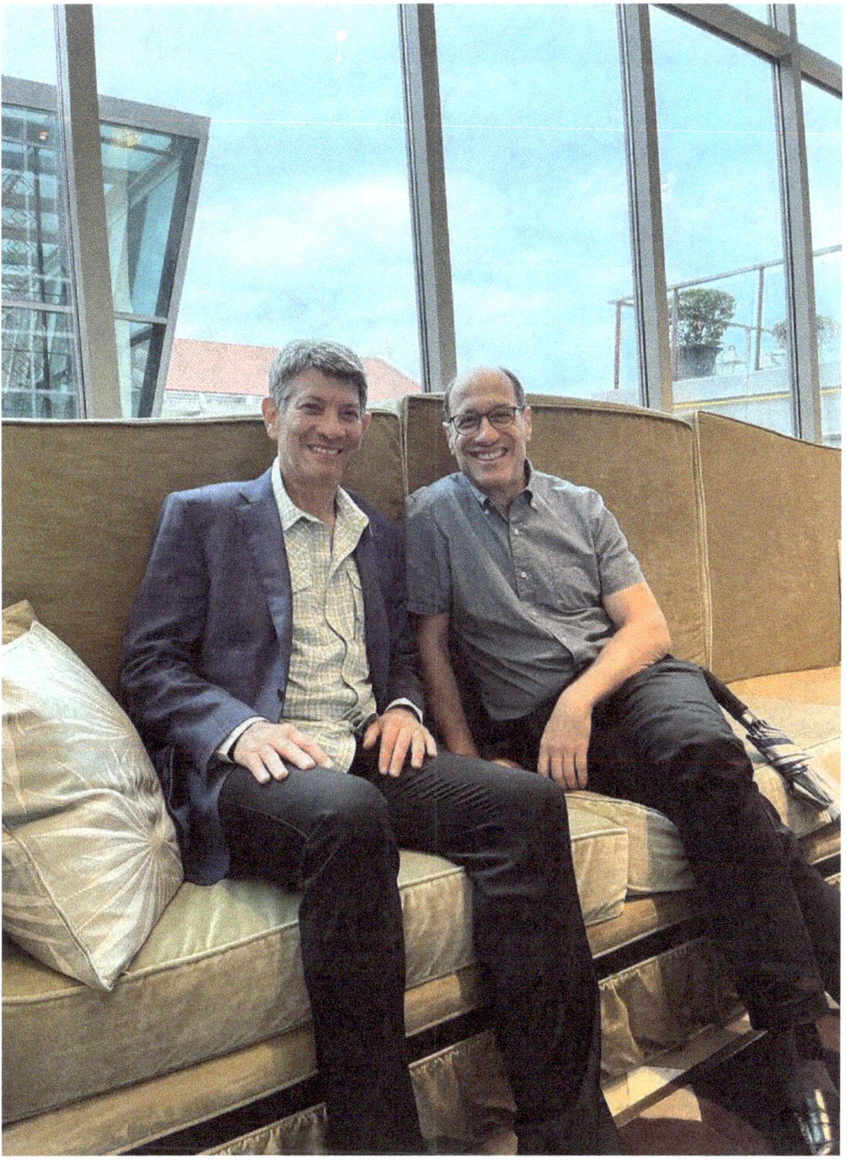

Prof David Allen and his eldest brother, Steven [Courtesy of Prof David Allen]

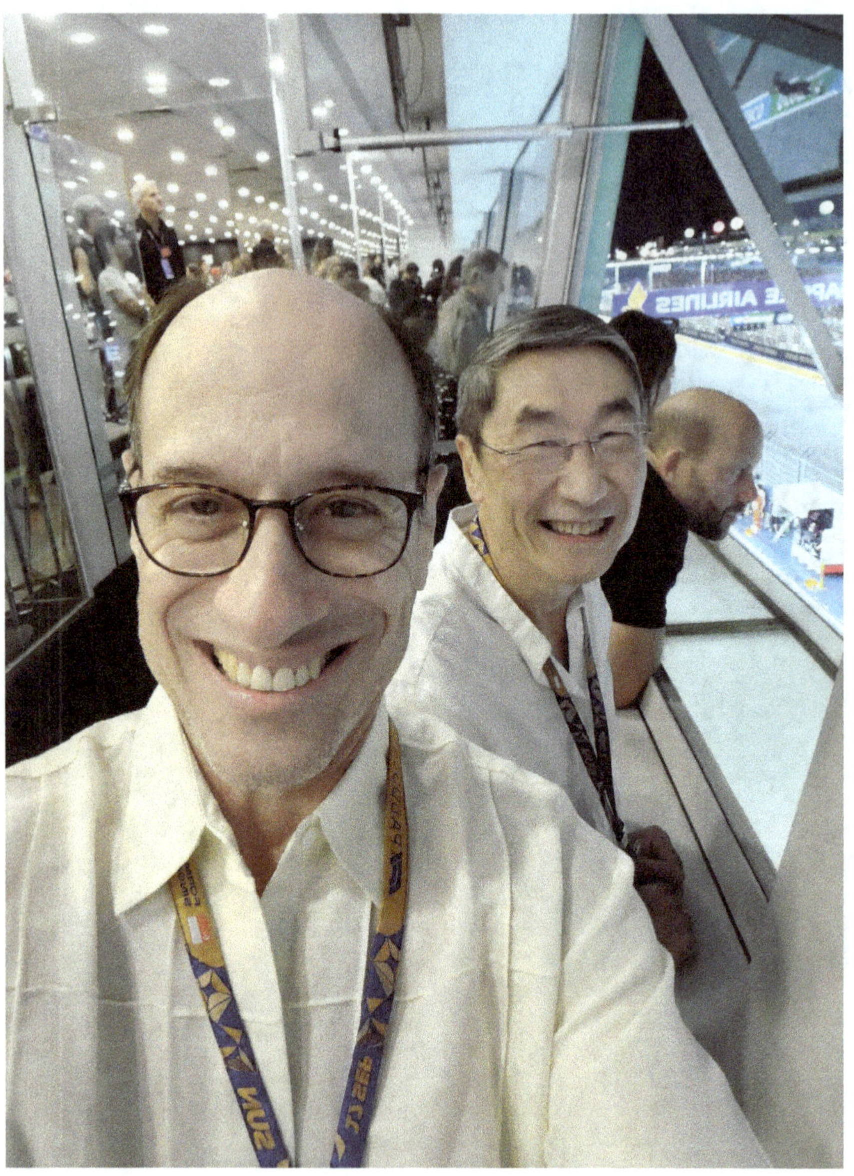

Old friends Prof David Allen and Prof John Wong at the Singapore Grand Prix, 2023
[Courtesy of Prof David Allen]

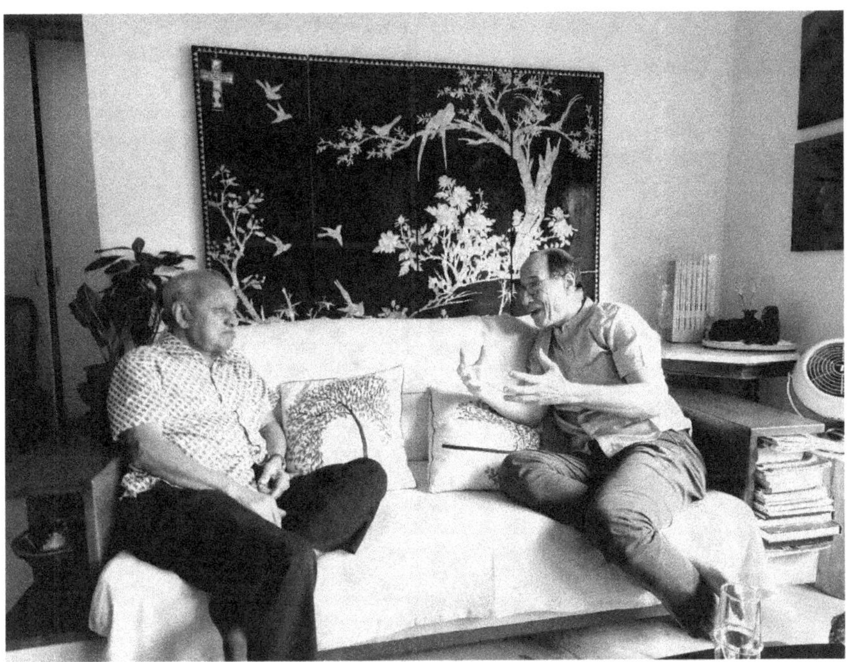

A catch-up between Dr Edmund Monteiro and Prof David Allen, 13 Apr 2024

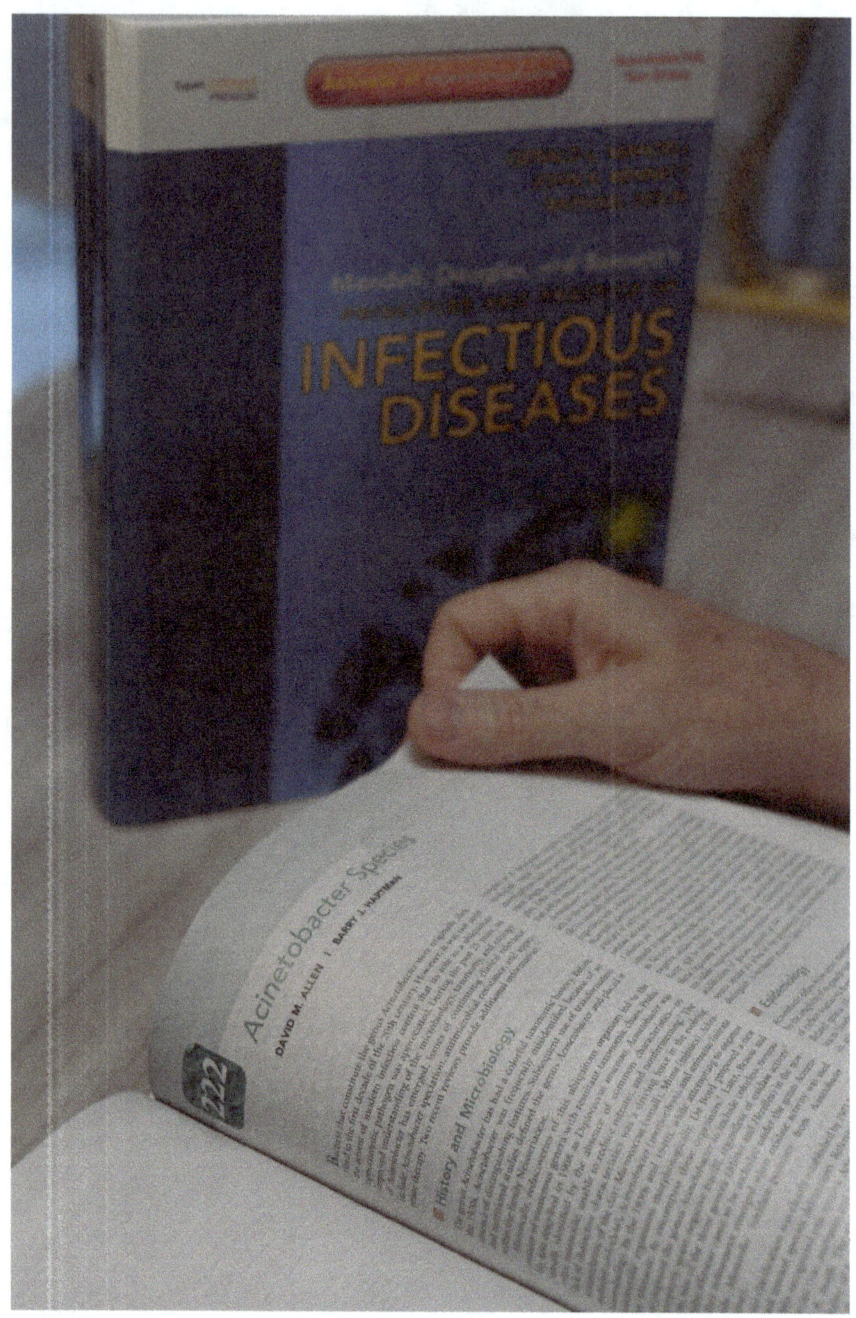

Chapter 222 of the Seventh Edition of Mandell, Douglas, and Bennett's Principles and Practice of Infectious Diseases, on the topic of '*Acinetobacter Species*', co-authored by Prof David Allen. [Photo by Dr Goh Yihui]

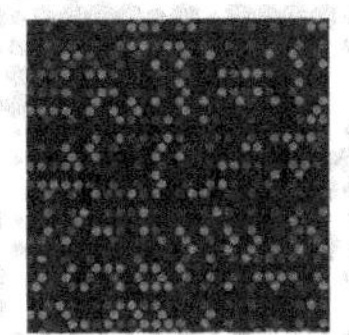

THE AUTHORS AND PHOTOGRAPHER

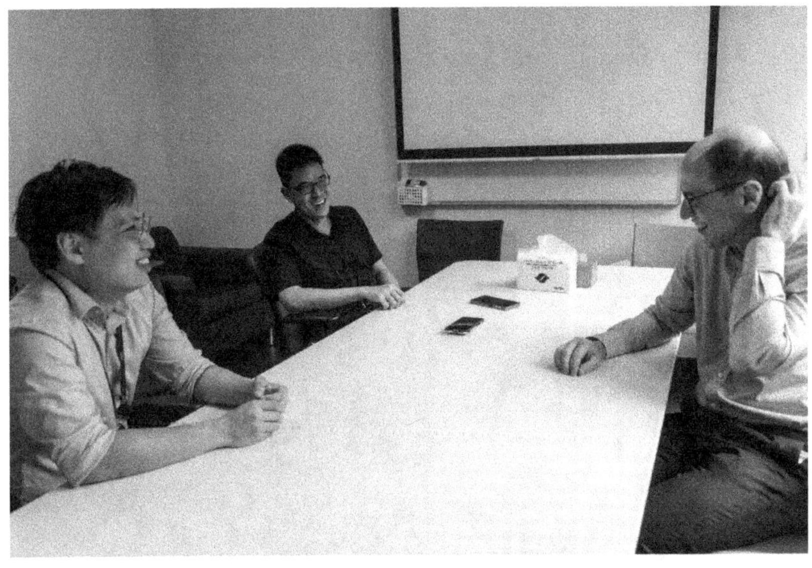

The final interview session
From left to right: Nicholas, Gabriel, and David

Nicholas is an infectious diseases physician working at the National University Hospital. He trained under the Internal Medicine and Infectious Diseases residency programme in NUH, where he first met Professor David Allen, became inspired by him and also inspired to share this narrative. Beyond a passion for ID, he enjoys downtime with family, friends and hobbies including reading fiction, watching serials and listening to podcasts on just about anything. The little remaining free time he has left is used to strongly implore Gab to read more fiction.

Gabriel is an infectious diseases physician and a clinical microbiologist who currently works at the National University Hospital as well as the National Public Health Laboratory. He is also an adjunct assistant professor with the National University of Singapore. He considers it his privilege to be able to pick the brains of, as well as banter with, Professor David Allen on countless occasions. He has a passion for collecting rare cases and pictures of pathogens that he comes across, and otherwise devotes his time to reading just about anything that interests him — mostly non-fiction, but has otherwise been persuaded by Nic to expand his range to fiction as well.

Yihui is a neurologist working at the National University Hospital who dabbles in photography in her non-existent free time. She worked with, and learnt much from Professor David Allen during the COVID-19 pandemic. Unfortunately, Gabriel feels she still has much to learn in terms of coming up with good ID puns.

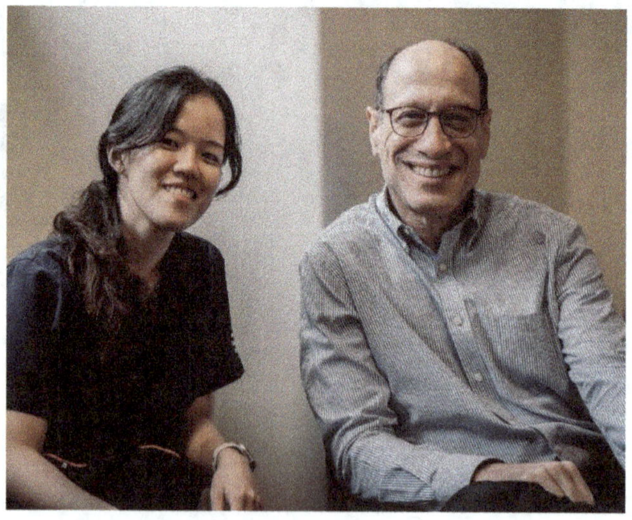

Photoshoot with the photographer — Yihui and David
Yihui is the cover and interview photoshoot photographer

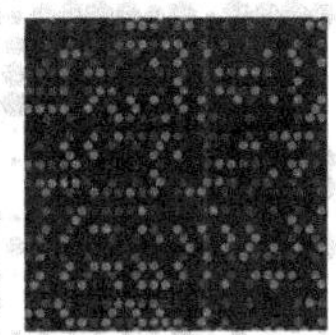

INDEX